"A rare combination of literary history and psychoanalysis, this book opens a thought-provoking perspective on Surrealism and psychoanalysis, poetry and dream analysis, through the work of Andreas Embiricos, Greece's first Surrealist poet and its first practicing psychoanalyst. A colleague of Jacques Lacan, Embiricos trained in Paris and remained close to Marie Bonaparte, Freud's key ally in France. His writings on Freudian psychoanalysis are marked by passion and a distinctive Surrealist imagination. This book offers two clinical cases that highlight his sensitive approach to dream work. A unique contribution to the literature, this book invites reflection on the practice of psychoanalysis today and may renew the analyst's capacity for free association."

Christine Anzieu-Premmereur, *Assistant Clinical Professor in Psychiatry at Columbia University, USA*

The Collected Psychoanalytic Writings of Andreas Embiricos

This book presents the psychoanalytic writings of the Greek Surrealist Andreas Embiricos in English for the first time.

A pioneer of psychoanalysis in Greece, Embiricos produced two remarkable case studies that highlight his unique practice of psychoanalysis, clinically rigorous and resolutely Surrealist in its belief in the revolutionary potentialities of Eros. The volume also includes a lecture on psychoanalytic technique from the 1940s, together with several texts on the life and work of Princess Marie Bonaparte, a close friend and collaborator of Embiricos. Complementing these writings are an interview in which Embiricos reflects on his psychoanalytic practice, and four scholarly essays examining key dimensions of his psychoanalytic career and intellectual legacy.

Bringing together clinical material, historical documents, and contemporary scholarship, this unique collection will be of interest to psychoanalysts as well as to scholars of the history of psychoanalysis, Surrealism, Greek literature, and European intellectual and cultural history.

Andreas Embiricos (1901–1975) was a Greek poet, writer, and psychoanalyst. He is recognized as one of the foremost Greek Surrealists and the first Freudian psychoanalyst in Greece.

Alexander Baron-Raiffe is a licensed psychoanalyst in private practice in New York City, USA.

The Collected Psychoanalytic Writings of Andreas Embiricos

Andreas Embiricos

Editor of the Greek edition

Giōrgos Kourias

Editor and Translator of the English edition

Alexander Baron-Raiffe

Routledge
Taylor & Francis Group
LONDON AND NEW YORK

ΜΙΑ ΠΕΡΙΠΤΩΣΙΣ ΙΔΕΟΨΥΧΑΝΑΓΚΑΣΤΙΚΗΣ ΝΕΥΡΩΣΕΩΣ ΜΕ ΠΡΟΩΡΕΣ ΕΚΣΠΕΡΜΑΤΩΣΕΙΣ ΚΑΙ ΑΛΛΑ ΨΥΧΑΝΑΛΥΤΙΚΑ ΚΕΙΜΕΝΑ

First published in English 2027
by Routledge
4 Park Square, Milton Park, Abingdon, Oxon OX14 4RN

and by Routledge
605 Third Avenue, New York, NY 10158

Routledge is an imprint of the Taylor & Francis Group, an informa business

Chapters 1, 2, 3, 4, 5, 7, 8, and 9 First Published in Greek by Agra as *Mia periptōsis ideopsychanagkastikēs neurōseōs me proōres ekspermatōseis kai alla psychanalytika keimena*

Chapter 6 First Published in Greek as: " 'Machomai dia tēn apeleutherōsin tou erōta.' Synenteuksē me ton A. Empeiriko." *Ēridanos*, no. 4, 1976.

Chapter 10 First Published in Greek as " ' . . .Opōs oles oi gynaikes oi omoies me autē, opōs ē Alkmēne . . .': Gynaikeia kai antrikē omophylophilia sto ergo tou Empeirikou." *Comparison / Comparaison / Sygkrisē*, no. 31, 2022.

Chapter 11 First Publihsed in Greek as "Maria Vonapartē kai Andreas Empeirikos: Ē aparches tēs psychanalysēs. Apo tēn euphoria stēn mataiōsē." *Ellēnikē Psychanalytikē Epitheōrēsē*, no. 1, 2025.

British Library Cataloguing-in-Publication Data
A catalogue record for this book is available from the British Library

ISBN: 978-1-041-12634-8 (hbk)
ISBN: 978-1-041-12633-1 (pbk)
ISBN: 978-1-003-66576-2 (ebk)

DOI: 10.4324/9781003665762

Typeset in Times New Roman
by Apex CoVantage, LLC

Contents

Translator's Acknowledgments

This translation is dedicated to the memory of my friend, Dr. Jared Russell, whose early encouragement first led me to consider translating Andreas Embiricos' psychoanalytic writings into English.

I wish to record my gratitude to Professor Efthymia Rentzou, who introduced me to Embiricos' work during my graduate studies at Princeton University. My fellowship at Princeton's Seeger Center for Hellenic Studies afforded me the opportunity to deepen my engagement with Modern Greek language and culture, ultimately making the present undertaking possible.

I am indebted to all of my dear friends in Greece, but especially to Mr. Orestis Andrianis and Ms. Phoebe Karvela who, recognizing my enthusiasm for Embiricos and the fact that I had recently begun psychoanalytic training at the time, thoughtfully presented me with a copy of his *Psychoanalytic Papers* in Greek as a birthday gift nearly a decade ago.

I extend my warmest thanks to Mr. Leonidas Embiricos and Mr. Stavros Petsopoulos for their trust in authorizing this translation, and to Ms. Sofia Bougioukli for her attentive reading and insightful edits of my translations from the Greek.

Finally, I thank Dr. Vaia Tsolas for her enthusiasm for this project and for graciously agreeing to write the Introduction.

Translator's Preface

Alexander Baron-Raiffe

Although renowned in his home country and acknowledged in Europe for the significance of his poetry within the Surrealist movement, Andreas Embiricos, Greece's first psychoanalyst and first Surrealist poet, remains little known in the Anglophone psychoanalytic and literary worlds.[1] Born in Brăila, Romania, in 1901 to a prominent Greek shipping family, Embiricos occupied, until his death in Athens in 1975, a singular position at the confluence of two of the twentieth century's most radical intellectual movements. Indeed, Embiricos was the only member of André Breton's Surrealist group to have also been a practicing psychoanalyst. Every translation inevitably involves a wish to bring an author's work to a broader audience. In the case of Andreas Embiricos, my aim is to invite contemporary psychoanalysts and scholars of intellectual history to discover a psychoanalytic and Surrealist pioneer from Greece—a nation that is culturally, geographically, and historically at both the heart of and the periphery of Europe.

Yet, to translate Embiricos is not merely to render accessible the writings of an "unknown" figure positioned at the margins of European psychoanalysis or Surrealism. It is also to illuminate an alternative trajectory that psychoanalysis itself might have taken, a speculative history of what a largely forgotten branch of Freudian psychoanalysis might have become had certain historical, personal, and theoretical contingencies unfolded differently—namely, an orthodox Freudianism inflected by Surrealism. While Jacques Lacan's distinctively Surrealist-tinged psychoanalysis is the best-known outcome of the encounter between psychoanalysis and surrealism, it was, as the present volume reveals, not the only one.[2] And unlike Lacan, Embiricos remained programmatically Surrealist throughout his career. The writings in this volume show that Embiricos felt no incompatibility between a rigorously Freudian clinical stance and a vision of psychoanalysis as endowed with profoundly revolutionary potential. This introduction therefore proposes that Embiricos should be read not as a neglected Greek Surrealist or a provincial Freudian, but rather as a figure whose life and work illuminate the intellectual ferment of interwar Paris, where reciprocal encounters between psychoanalysis and Surrealism engendered a distinct form of psychoanalysis, saturated with poetic and revolutionary energy: a distinctly Surrealist psychoanalysis.

Embiricos, traveling frequently between Paris and Athens, participated in many of the significant intellectual fora of the interwar period that would continue to shape both French intellectual life and psychoanalysis after the Second World War.[3] In 1933, he was introduced to André Breton by his friend Jean-Frois Wittmann, and he formally joined the Place Blanche Surrealist Group in 1935.[4] There, beyond Breton, he formed close ties with Paul Éluard, Yves Tanguy, and Óscar Dominguez.[5] During this same period, he also attended Alexandre Kojève's epochal lectures on Hegel alongside Jacques Lacan.[6] Also in 1935, in Athens, he introduced Surrealism to the Greek public in a landmark lecture [*Peri Sourrealismou*] at the Artists' Club, published *Blast Furnace* [*Hypsikaminos*] (the first collection of Surrealist poetry in the Greek language), and became the first IPA-affiliated analyst to open a psychoanalytic practice in Greece.

After the end of the Second World War, he remained in Greece until 1951, when pressure from the conservative medical establishment forced him to close his analytic practice. Although he continued as a member and training analyst of the *Société psychanalytique de Paris* (SPP) until the early 1960s and maintained a keen interest in psychoanalysis until his death in 1975, he never again practiced clinically. After the closure of his practice, he spent several years in Paris and dedicated himself exclusively to literature and photography for the remainder of his life.[7] He continued to take trips to Western Europe, maintained a correspondence with André Breton until at least 1958,[8] and kept himself abreast of developments in psychoanalysis; yet he never returned to clinical work or psychoanalytic writing.

In this sense, one may say that the War, and the conservative and repressive forces in Greece and elsewhere, claimed Andreas Embiricos' psychoanalytic career as one of their victims. In the upheavals of the mid-twentieth century, the revolutionary ambitions that had electrified the followers of both psychoanalysis and Surrealism were sharply curtailed.[9] What had once appeared as intellectual praxes based on abstract, universal, and theoretical thinking capable of transforming the human condition gradually gave way—whether through cooptation by the medical establishment, institutional and intellectual conservatism, or theoretical shifts—to more adaptative, developmental, and "scientific," "observational," or "objective" paradigms. Surrealism, born of Freud's discovery of the sexual unconscious, aspired to mobilize artistic and literary creation to produce a collective encounter with unconscious desire—one powerful enough to transform social, political, economic, and sexual life.[10] The ambition that psychoanalysis could accomplish the same through individual cures, free clinics, educational establishments, and social reform, also faded away in the post-War years.

Embiricos' lecture on psychoanalytic technique (Chapter 3 of this volume) is the only surviving text in which he explicitly formulates his clinical orientation. It reveals a striking synthesis, even perhaps a paradox: a rigorously orthodox analytic frame (preliminary interviews, fixed session times six days a week, classical neutrality, use of the couch, payment of the fee, etc.) combined with a revolutionary vision in which the analyst becomes at once "trainer of the liberated revolutionary forces" and "disciplined and aware agent provocateur." Even so, the analyst must remain entirely neutral regarding the aims toward which the patient deploys the newly liberated quantity of libidinal energy. His intellectual fidelity to Freud is likewise evident in the two case studies included in this volume. Across these writings, Freud's project and Breton's appear not as antagonistic but as mutually reinforcing: the psychoanalyst and the Surrealist emerge as twin figures in a shared struggle against repression.

This dynamic is already visible in his 1935 lecture *On Surrealism* [*Peri Sourrealismou*], where Embiricos compares Freud's discovery of the unconscious to Columbus's discovery of the New World.[11] The Surrealist poem, he argued, is a dream in waking life freed from the prohibitions of the superego.[12] In his intellectual pantheon, Freud and Breton are celebrated as liberators of desire, each confirming the other's discoveries: Freud establishes the universality of the unconscious, Surrealism affords the means for its deployment.[13] "Surrealism," he wrote, offers

> the possibility of the direct use of the potentiality of the psyche in its purest and most unadulterated form, a possibility that guarantees, more than any other attempt known to date, the fullest possible emancipation of the spiritual human being from the inhuman and perverse codes of unnatural moral and aesthetic codes imposed upon our sensibility.[14]

This mirrors André Breton's own formulation:

> Surrealism is based on the belief in the superior reality of certain forms of previously neglected associations, in the omnipotence of dream, in the disinterested play of thought. It tends to ruin once and for all all other psychic mechanisms and to substitute itself for them in solving all the principal problems of life.[15]

What would it mean today for psychoanalysts to once again grant the neglected productions of psychic life such an exalted place, to conceive analytic practice itself as a form of lived poetry?

Embiricos' revolutionary optimism in Surrealism was not unique. Walter Benjamin, writing in 1929, observed:

> Since Bakunin, Europe has lacked a radical concept of freedom. The Surrealists have one. They are the first to liquidate the sclerotic moral-humanistic ideal of freedom, because they are convinced that "freedom, which on this earth can only be bought with a thousand of the hardest sacrifices, must be

> enjoyed unrestrictedly in its fullness without any sort of pragmatic calculation, as long as it lasts."[16]

These lines could well have been written by Embiricos. For him, psychoanalysis was Surrealism by another name: an organized system for countering repression in all of its forms.

To contemporary readers, such an idea may appear naïve or utopian, yet I would suggest that Embiricos' synthesis of Freudian orthodoxy and revolution is of particular relevance to the present day, given the repressive, totalitarian, and sanguinary forces at work in the world. At a moment when Freudian psychoanalysis is often dismissed as rigid, intellectualizing, outdated, or even complicit in repression—especially where questions of gender, sexuality, and "identity" are concerned—Embiricos' writings remind us that another configuration once existed, and may still be thinkable: a psychoanalysis conceived as a theory and praxis of radical freedom, one capable of discerning the forces that constrain desire in ever-new guises, whether social, political, identitarian, or technological. In doing so, Embiricos unsettles several assumptions that have become almost axiomatic in contemporary Anglo-American analytic discourse, assumptions that tend to draw clinical practice away from its foundations in metapsychological inquiry and toward a clinic centered on concepts such as affect, attunement, or empathy.

In broad outline, this discourse often portrays classical Freudian psychoanalysis—frequently conflated in American contexts with ego-psychology—as limited by its metapsychological assumptions and its emphasis on the Oedipus and on sexuality, allegedly at the expense of more "primitive" psychic processes. Closely related is the conviction that analytic treatment depends above all on flexibility, emotional responsiveness, and empathic validation. In contrast, neutrality, a stable analytic frame, and an interpretative, non-gratifying stance are viewed as risks for retraumatization, despite their grounding in a Freudian theory of the unconscious. Indeed, theory, in this perspective, is best kept secondary to practice; instinct, affect, and responsiveness are taken as the clinician's primary guides (often subsumed under the heading "counter-transference"), and the analyst's task is increasingly framed as affirming the patient's identities, narratives, and sense of self. In other words, affect is the royal road to an unconscious that is altogether too reassuring and too conscious to bear much resemblance at all to anything like Freud's radical, disquieting, scandalous, and uncanny unconscious.

Although my presentation of these positions is of course schematic and by no means universally endorsed, they are sufficiently widespread to render the paradox at the heart of Embiricos' work especially provocative for contemporary analysts. How, and why, did a radical Surrealist poet—who nonetheless identified himself as an orthodox Freudian—find in a form of theory and clinical practice now often dismissed as rigid or intellectualizing the very conditions for psychic and political liberation? Even if the case studies collected in this volume are not to be taken as models for contemporary psychoanalytic practice, they nonetheless invite us to resist the reflexive turn away from abstraction, general theorization, and speculative thought. In doing so, they challenge us to reconsider whether the eclipse of Freudian metapsychology may also entail the loss of a more radical imagination—one oriented toward liberation from the repressive tedium of the conscious and the quotidian forms of constraint it quietly sustains.

The texts published in this book testify to the profound continuity between Embiricos' analytic and literary writing, in which sexuality, fantasy, and revolt against hypocrisy, mediocrity, and the repressive *status quo* form an interlocking whole. Although little of his literary work has been translated into English, complicating access for non-Greek-speaking scholars, the writings gathered in the present volume provide insight into his metapsychology.[17] They show the great importance for Embiricos of the primal scene, the structuring function of identifications in psychic life, the enduring centrality of polymorphous and infantile sexuality throughout life, and the drive toward sexual and artistic ecstasy.[18]

To read Embiricos today is thus to encounter a lost possibility within Freudian thought: a psychoanalysis that perceived no incompatibility between an austerely orthodox frame and an avant-garde revolutionary praxis—one that regarded itself as contiguous with poetry, and one that centered Eros as a force of transformation and life. His writings demonstrate the contributions that lay analysts can make to psychoanalysis, and the capacity of analytic theory and clinical practice to explore forms of desire in which the linguistic and the libidinal, the practical and the aspirational, the psychic and the somatic, and the political and the personal remain inseparably intertwined.

The papers in this volume restore to view a thinker for whom the analytic and the surreal were never opposites, but dual expressions of the same desire: to bring to light what is repressed, to give form to the formless, words to the ineffable, and to imagine, however fleetingly, a New World.

Notes

1 For a general account of the history of psychoanalysis in Greece, see: Danae Karydaki, "Freud Under the Acropolis: The Challenging Journey of Psychoanalysis in 20th-Century Greece (1915–1995)," *History of the Human Sciences* 31, no. 4 (2018): 13–37; Anna Potamianou, "Greece," in *International Dictionary of Psychoanalysis*, ed. Alain de Mijolla (New York: Macmillan, 2005), 700–1.

2 On Lacan's engagement with the Surrealists, see: David Macey, *Lacan in Contexts* (New York: Verso, 1988). See also: Elisabeth Roudinesco, *Jacques Lacan: histoire d'une vie, esquisse d'un système de pensée* (Paris: Fayard, 1993).

3 For a full account of Embiricos' psychoanalytic career, see Chapters 8 and 11; Andreas Embiricos, "Tēlegraphēma pros André Breton," *Delear* no. 3 (June 2001): 12.

4 Andreas Embiricos, "Tēlegraphēma pros André Breton," *Delear* no. 3 (June 2001): 12.
5 Nikos Sigalas, *Ho Andreas Empeirikos kai hē historia tou hellēnikou hyperrealismou ē brosta stēn ameiliktē archē tēs pragmatikotētas* (Athens: Agra, 2012), 91ff, cited in Helena Badell Giralt, "Salvador Dalí i el surrealisme grec," *Revue d'Études Catalanes* no. 3 (2018): 70–9, 76.
6 Badell Giralt, "Salvador Dalí i el surrealisme grec," 70–79, 76.
7 Embiricos' remarkable photographic work has been published in two monographs: *Phōtophraktēs: hē phōtographies tou Andrea Empeirikou* (Athens: Agra, 2001) and *Hē Andros tou Andrea Empeirikou* (Athens: Agra, 2004). It was also featured in the exhibition "Surrealism Beyond Borders," *Metropolitan Museum of Art*, New York, 4 October 2021–30 January 2022, and a recent exhibition entitled "Andreas Embiricos: Photographs Never Shown Before" at the Eleftheria Tseliou Gallery, Athens, 3 June–12 September 2025.
8 Andreas Empeirikos, "Gramma ston André Breton," *Outopia* no. 49 (March–April 2002): 45.
9 Laurence Kahn has shown how it is especially abstract, metapsychological thinking that did not survive the intellectual persecutions of the Nazi regime. See: *What Nazism Did to Psychoanalysis* (Abington, Oxon: Routledge, 2022).
10 For an excellent general reference on Surrealism's theoretical foundations, see: Jennifer Mundy (ed.), *Surrealism: Desire Unbound* (Princeton, NJ: Princeton University Press, 2001); see also: Hal Foster, *Compulsive Beauty* (Cambridge, MA: MIT Press, 1993).
11 Andreas Empeirikos, *Peri Sourrealismou: Hē Dialexē tou 1935* (Athens: Agra, 2009), 69. All translations mine. The metaphor of the New World will be central to Embiricos' magnum opus, the novel *The Great Eastern* [*Ho Megas Anatolikos*].
12 Empeirikos, *Peri Sourrealismou*, 72–73. Athens, Greece: AGRA Publications.
13 Empeirikos, *Peri Sourrealismou*, 75–76. Athens, Greece: AGRA Publications.
14 Empeirikos, *Peri Sourrealismou*, 77. Athens, Greece: AGRA Publications.
15 *Manifestos of Surrealism*, trans. Richard Seaver and Helen R. Lane (Ann Arbor, MI: University of Michigan Press, 1969), 24.
16 Walter Benjamin, "Surrealism: The Last Snapshot of the European Intelligentsia," trans. Edmond Jephcott, *New Left Review* no. 108 (1978): 47–56, 54.
17 In English, the only volume of poetry to have been translated is: *Amour Amour*, trans. Nikos Stangos and Alan Ross (København and Los Angeles: Green Integer, 2003). Various poems by Embiricos have been published in literary journals and anthologies.
18 One possible avenue of further study would be the extent to which Embiricos' views on infantile sexuality were influenced by those of his friend and mentor, Marie Bonaparte. On this subject, see: Constantin Makris, "Roman surréaliste et écriture 'auto-analytique': Le 'Great Eastern' d'Andréas Embiricos," *Mélusine* no. 26 (2006): 257–74. Nikos Sigalas' essay, published as Chapter 10 of the present volume, is an important contribution to understanding Embiricos' views on homosexuality.

A Note on the English Translation

This book includes all of the material that was originally published in French and Greek in the 2001 volume edited by Giōrgos Kourias and published by Ekdoseis Agra in Athens. I have added three chapters to the present English edition, which together offer a fuller picture of Andreas Embiricos the psychoanalyst—how he worked, thought, and conceptualized his clinical vocation. These include: Chapter 6, a 1967 interview conducted by Andromachē Skarpalezou in Paris, the only instance in which Embiricos spoke publicly about his psychoanalytic practice; Chapter 10, a recent article by Nikos Sigalas concerning Embiricos' views on homosexuality; and Chapter 11, an essay by his son, Leōnidas Embiricos, which draws on recently discovered archival material to illuminate not only Embiricos' close professional and personal relationship with Princess Marie Bonaparte, but also their sustained efforts to establish an official psychoanalytic society in Greece after the Second World War.

Regarding the romanization of Greek in the text, all Greek words and names romanized in the main text and footnotes follow the American Library Association–Library of Congress (ALA-LC) guidelines for the romanization of Greek. The principal exception is the name Embiricos, for which the older French romanization preferred by the author has been retained in the main text. However, where his name appears bibliographical references romanized from Greek in the footnotes, his name appears as *Empeirikos* following ALA-LC standards.

Editor's Preface to the Greek Edition

Giōrgos Kourias

The magnitude of Andreas Embiricos' poetic presence in Greek letters has, perhaps inevitably, left his psychoanalytic identity and activity somewhat in the shadows. And yet, these formed a significant part of his life, and his interest in Freud's work, and in the developments in the psychoanalytic world more broadly, appears to have continued unabated even after he ceased clinical practice around 1951.

It is true that, in comparison with his literary corpus (both poetry and prose), his published or otherwise known psychoanalytic writings appear sparse. But we should be cautious about drawing hasty conclusions regarding a corresponding lack of engagement. We might instead consider that, because of the uniquely extroverted nature of literary expression, whereas a poet exists only in relationship to his real or imagined readership, Embiricos the psychoanalyst was oriented toward the inner world of his private office and toward the daily construction (except Sunday, as we will read!) of an "analytic space" with his patients—a space that by its nature resists disclosure.

The psychoanalytic work of Andreas Embiricos cannot fail to be of particular interest to the Greek analytic community, since he is recognized as the first Greek psychoanalyst. It was he who first introduced Freudianism to Greece as a theory and a clinical practice. Yet even the non-specialist reader may find compelling interest in this testimony of the work and thought of a man who, within a Greek society that was completely hostile to the influence of psychoanalysis—at a time in which such influence was spreading through the medical and intellectual landscapes of Europe—dedicated himself, in solitude, to the service of a science that he believed would fundamentally transform the world.

Thus, we decided to publish in this volume the psychoanalytic writings of Andreas Embiricos. Among them, the lengthy clinical monograph "A Case of Obsessional Neurosis with Premature Ejaculations," published in 1950 in the *Revue Française de Psychanalyse*, stands out. More complete than all the other existing texts, it is naturally this one which, precisely because of its completeness, lends itself to critical analysis—an analysis which it was written to invite.

The three other texts that follow are unpublished and were found in the poet's archives. The first of them, "A Case of Unconscious Homosexuality," is a half-completed report—at least in the version that was found—also in French, of another psychoanalytic treatment conducted by Embiricos. It is followed by the transcription of a talk he gave, again in French, on the topic of psychoanalytic technique. From the context, it can be inferred that it forms part of a series of talks he gave to an audience not specialized in psychoanalysis. As to where and when (and whether) the talks in question may have been given, no information is available that would allow us to give an answer. It is nonetheless reasonable to assume that this particular text dates back to the 1940s or the early 1950s.

The manuscript, unfortunately, breaks off abruptly, and so we only possess a portion of this particular lecture. Nonetheless, the interest it holds is, I believe, twofold. On the one hand, since it sets forth his views on analytic technique, it offers a glimpse into how Embiricos the psychoanalyst worked. Viewed in light of this lecture, the treatment of Giannis T. in the lengthy case study I referenced earlier becomes, for the informed reader, immediately more revealing with regard to what transpired between analyst and patient. On the other hand, because during the same period—as Thanasēs Tsavaras explains in his related article, included in this volume—efforts were underway to secure recognition from the International Psychoanalytic Association for the first psychoanalytic group that formed in Greece around Embiricos, the lecture offers the valuable opportunity to assess of the level of psychoanalytic discourse among those who were its natural—and officially recognized—representatives in Greece.

The cycle ends with the unpublished text "In Memory of Marie Bonaparte." This manuscript was written in Greek, and it was found amongst the papers of the poet who apparently wrote it in 1963. It consists of a posthumous encomium to the Princess and a biographical note on the life and work of this woman who played such an important role in Andreas Embiricos' relationship to psychoanalysis.

I want to thank Mrs. Vivika Embiricou and Mr. Leonidas Embiricos for the trust they showed in this undertaking, granting us access to the poet's unpublished writings and offering invaluable help through their information and guidance.

Introduction to the English Edition

Vaia Tsolas

A striking feature of Embiricos's psychoanalytic writings is his emphasis on the orthodoxy of Freudian discoveries about drives and the unconscious, particularly the centrality of sexuality. A Surrealist poet, Embiricos was eager to introduce Freudian revolutionary discoveries to his home country of Greece, and the path he chose was to challenge the resistance by remaining steadfastly loyal to the Freudian text. Consequently, Embiricos affords the contemporary reader a unique opportunity to witness the significant contrast between what psychoanalysis was in the poet's time and what it is today.

In this brief introduction, I highlight the prevalence of language related to sexuality and the body and, in that, propose that Embiricos offers a pathway to rediscover psychosexuality, to inhabit a world of paradox where meaning is continuously created and found via the language of the body that is the bedrock of the psyche.

I don't discuss here the historical underpinnings of the shift in psychoanalysis away from the centrality of sexuality toward the object, a topic that has been widely discussed, debated, and displayed throughout a plethora of psychoanalytic writings. Andre Green, in his article "Has Sexuality Anything to Do with Psychoanalysis?" succinctly and pointedly describes this contemporary undermining of sexuality as either biological or old-fashioned when he says:

> It [sexuality] is no longer considered to be a major factor in child development nor an aetiological determinant for the understanding of clinical psychopathology. It is as if sexuality were now considered a topic of specialised significance, a limited area of the internal world among other such.[1]

The meaning and function Freud endowed it with in his work seem to be almost entirely lost, Green suggests. Green points out that the entire theory of the drives has been discredited and devalued: "This even went as far as the interpretation of material in which the sexual was manifestly visible as a form of defence against anxieties or regressions, allegedly situated at a more archaic level."[2]

Embiricos not only returns sexuality and the drives to their central position as the basis and support of the psyche, but also clearly demonstrates through his own work the manner in which Freud constructed his revolutionary psychoanalytic method on the foundation of his discovery of sexuality as the etiology of neurosis. In his clinical work, Embiricos elegantly forwards his fluency in the language of dreams to equate them with the language of symptoms, both rooted entirely in sexuality and the body.

Many decades later, Didier Anzieu's work was devoted entirely to the idea that the unconscious is structured like the body, contrasting Lacan's proposition that the unconscious is structured like a language. Anzieu writes:

> The unconscious seems to me to be structured like the body—not the body as studied and represented by anatomo-physiologists, but the body of the phantastic anatomy of hysteria and infantile sexual theories (as Freud clearly showed); and, more fundamentally still, in a more primary and archaic manner, the body as source of the first sensory-motor experiences, the first communications, and the oppositions that relate to the very basis perception and thought.[3]

I propose that this primary, archaic language of sensorimotoreality is inherently steeped in paradox, as are the drives and the unconscious. In my opinion, much trouble in psychoanalytic theorizing stems from moving away from this paradoxical paradigm and attempting to resolve it by leaning either toward the physical, anatomical concrete body or toward the disembodied mind and language.

As a poet immersed in the language of the primary process, Embiricos plays and speaks to his patients through these paradoxes of a sexual language. This language does not ask to be resolved and dissolved in dichotomies of meaning, neither concrete genitalia nor abstract metaphors. The contemporary reader, in their own resistance to dwell in the paradox of the sexual, might appreciate the resistance Embiricos encountered among his contemporaries.

Embiricos recognizes this clearly—in his interview with Skarpalezou (Chapter 6), Embiricos writes, "Many of my writings have not been published. Because of how libertine they are. They offend polite ears." This is similar to Freud's 1896 comment about the discovery of the cause of neurosis being infantile sexuality: "I understood that from that point on, I was one of those who had 'disturbed the sleep of the world,' as Hebbel says, and that I could not expect objectivity or tolerance."[4]

Despite obstacles and repercussions, Embiricos, whether he was working with his patients' resistances or conversing with his contemporaries in the oppressive, bourgeois Athenian society of his era, did not shy away from pushing Freud's discoveries forward with the hope of bringing enlightenment. "I repeat: I am fighting for an absolute freedom of thought and life. For the liberation of Eros."

Even picking random examples in Embiricos' detailed work of dream interpretation, it is not hard to demonstrate the paradox in Eros revealed in dreams and to show how similar it is to the paradox in poetry.

> The cigarette that Petros smokes symbolizes both the maternal breast and the penis. I explained to him that he treats the breast like a penis not only because he wishes to obtain gratification from both, but also because he seeks to compensate for the anxiety-inducing absence of a virile organ in his mother (whom he regards as having been castrated by his father) by imaginatively endowing her with one.
>
> p. 44

This passage very easily might be received by the reader as assigning old-fashioned psychoanalytic jargon to the patient's speech, the language of the period when Freud and his contemporaries struggled to make psychoanalysis a scientific method. However, readers need only consider the guiding principle of the drives—

> on the frontier between the mental and the somatic, as the psychical representative of the stimuli originating from within the organism and reaching the mind, as a measure of the demand made upon the mind for work in consequence of its connection with the body[5]

—to appreciate that this criticism overlooks the fact that psychoanalysis is carefully positioned by its creator at intersections of some/body/mind and filled with the richness of dynamic tensions.

In highlighting Freudian clinical practice, Embiricos rigorously follows a multitude of foundational psychoanalytic concepts: infantile sexuality being defined as a perverse sexuality with multiple possibilities for pleasure, psychosexuality not biologically determined but rather formed through identifications and conflicts in the Oedipus complex, and the subject being determined by both libidinous and destructive drives, are only a few of these psychoanalytic concepts. If the contemporary reader can tolerate this paradoxical language of metapsychology, and specifically that of psychosexuality, they may even be able to find the maddening quality of the unconscious in its poetic obscurity.

The cigarette, the maternal breast, and the penis all hold similar significance, yet they neither have nor lack their designated meaning. At the same time, their symbolic significance allows them to stand in for one another at the intersection of soma-libidinal body-unconscious fantasy, eliminating the need to resolve the paradox.

Embiricos continues:

> In this way, he expresses, alongside his desire to enjoy both the penis and the breast, the wish to restore his mother (and, through his identification with her, to restore himself) by conceiving of the breasts as possessing, in

> addition to their natural meaning as feminine attributes, a phallic or masculine significance . . . By smoking the cigarette, that is by sucking at the breast-penis, Petros let fall (or flow) onto his clothing the ash-milk-semen.
>
> p. 44

We hear the poet in the psychoanalyst here and what poetry can teach us about the paradox inherent in Freud's sexual language of drives and the unconscious.

Embiricos's poem of the Caryatids, which follows, perhaps can clue us in to the common language of the paradox inherent in both psychoanalysis and poetry.

O the breasts of youth
O the pallid waters of the fig-eaters
. . .
Youth senses your significance
And springs up already at your edges
Feathery tresses frisk between the breasts of young girls
Who walk half-naked through your narrow streets
Their curls more lovely than those of Absalom
. . .
The day sighs
One of the young daughters is playing with her breasts
No slap will do any good
A deer passes by holding in its mouth
The three cherries it found between the breasts of youth
The evening here is warm
The trees wrap themselves in their quietude
Now and then rocks of silence fall slowly into the clearing
Like light before it turns to day.[6]

The language of poetry is undoubtedly structured like the erogenous body, where internal and external boundaries blur. This structuring demands that the mind reorganize the chaos of experience in order to find the object, not just repair it (as some post-Kleinian theory might indicate). However, this finding is not a simple finding, but rather an arrival at "where we started and know the place for the first time."[7]

Winnicott's 1971 work on transitional phenomena and the intermediate area inherent in creative process highlights the immense significance of tolerating paradox. In the area of psychic functioning, he says, what is involved is essentially "the paradox and the acceptance of the paradox: the baby creates the object, but the object was there waiting to be created and to become a cathected object."[8]

Marion Milner, in her 1950 book *Not Being Able to Paint*, speaks of the creative process as one to be able to break down the barrier of space between self and other, yet at the same time to be able to maintain it. This seems to her to be the paradox of creativity.

> Since this inner life is the life of a body, with all its complexities of rhythms, tensions, releases, movement, balance, and taking up room in space, so surely the essential thing about the symbols is that they should show in themselves, through their formal pattern, a similar theme of structural tensions and balances and release, but transfigured into a timeless visual co-existence.[9]

Milner suggests this in what might have been a commentary on Embiricos's psychoanalytic language.

The artist, she continues, among other things, makes available for recall and contemplation what he feels are the most valuable moments of his psychophysical experience. In other words, the experience of the artist is an undifferentiated psychosomatic experience.

Milner states that in his concern for the permanence and immortality of his work, the artist seeks not only to defy his own mortality, as analysts have said, but also to convey the sense of timelessness that accompanies those moments: "He does in fact make tabernacles to house the spirit, with the result that others can share in his experiences, and he himself can have a permanent record of them after the high moment of transfiguration has passed."[10]

According to Milner, the artistic expression is in incarnated symbols that capture "the astounding experience of how it feels to be alive, the experience known from inside, of being a moving, living body in space, with capacities to relate oneself to other objects in space."[11] We see this clearly in the fluid imagery of "the breast" in Embiricos's poem.

Both poets and psychoanalysts—or, in the case of Embiricos, the poet-psychoanalyst—live, breathe, and create in a world of paradox. When working in the transference, Winnicott tells us, the analyst and patient are part of a larger process in the clinical setting in which the other is being continuously "created" and "found." Immersion in the transference experience requires suspending secondary processes and giving way to the primary processes of the body and sexuality, while maintaining the "as if" quality of this surrender. The challenge of sustaining this paradox is the canvas surrealistically painted in the creative process of analysis.

This is why Winnicott highlights the curious fact that, although psychoanalysts are accustomed to working with paradox in their clinical practice of transference and dreams, they may be resistant to the paradox in the language of sexuality and the body in theorizing. Winnicott, in his appraisal of Milner's *On Not Being Able to Paint*, notes that like people living in the arts, psychoanalysts in practice, all of whom "traffic in illusion" might be resistant to see that subjectivity based on wish fulfillment is the basis of objectivity when it comes to their theories.

Through his analytic journey as a faithful disciple of Freud, Embiricos presents us the venue to linger in the penumbral paradox of Freudian psychosexuality "like light before it turns to day."

Notes

1 André Green, "Has Sexuality Anything to Do with Psychoanalysis?," *The International Journal of Psychoanalysis* 76, no. 5 (1995): 871–83, at 871.
2 André Green, *The Chains of Eros: The Sexual in Psychoanalysis* (Abingdon: Routledge, 2018), 5, Kindle edition.
3 Didier Anzieu, *A Skin for Thought: Interviews with Gilbert Tarrab on Psychology and Psychoanalysis*, trans. Daphne Nash Briggs (London: Karnac, 1990), 43, Kindle edition.
4 Sigmund Freud, "Letter from Freud to Fleiss, April 26, 1896," in *The Complete Letters of Sigmund Freud to Wilhelm Fliess, 1887–1904*, trans. Jeffrey Masson (Cambridge, MA: Belknap, 1985), 184.
5 Sigmund Freud, "Instincts and Their Vicissitudes," in *The Standard Edition of the Complete Psychological Works of Sigmund Freud*, vol. 14, ed. and trans. James Strachey (London: Hogarth, 1957), 109–40, at 122.
6 Andreas Embiricos, "Caryatids," in *A Century of Greek Poetry: 1900–2000*, trans. Karen Emmeric (New York: Cosmos, 2004).
7 T. S. Eliot, *Four Quartets* (Eastbourne: Gardners, 2001).
8 D. W. Winnicott, *Playing and Reality* (London: Routledge, 2005), 89, Kindle edition.
9 Marion Milner, *On Not Being Able to Paint* (London: Routledge, 2010), 82, Kindle edition.
10 Marion Milner, *On Not Being Able to Paint* (London: Routledge, 2010), 83.
11 Marion Milner, *On Not Being Able to Paint* (London: Routledge, 2010), 83.

Part I

The Psychoanalytic Writings of Andreas Embiricos

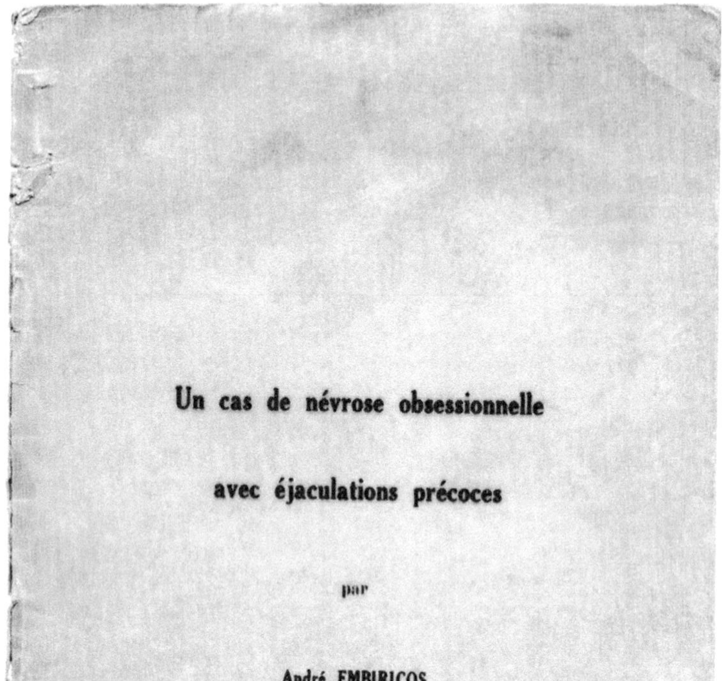

Figure 1.1 The cover of the offprint of the *Revue Française de Psychanalyse* in which the study "A Case of Obsessional Neurosis with Premature Ejaculation" was first published in French, in 1950.

Chapter 1

A Case of Obsessional Neurosis With Premature Ejaculation[1]

Giannis T. is the younger son of a rich merchant who, despite being a strict and authoritarian man, was very fond of his children. The patient came to consult me on his own initiative at the age of 29, for premature ejaculation and obsessional symptoms, which he himself recognized as such after having read several of Freud's works. He added that he has been masturbating since his tenderest youth, and that he still frequently indulges in onanism.

The patient's mother died when he was nine. Although he had been a delicate boy until the age of 12 or 13, he later grew into a robust and strong young man who enjoyed excellent health from a physical standpoint. He specifies that although he ejaculates prematurely, this only occurs with prostitutes, servant girls, and women of the lower classes; with women and young girls of his own social class, he is totally impotent. He noticed the latter phenomenon at the age of 21, following an attempt at coitus with a young female university student who had awakened feelings of love in him, and after three subsequent attempts at coitus two years later with a divorced lady who was attracted to him, and had done everything to seduce him, taking the initiative herself in all of the games of love.

He also tells me that, where women are concerned, he had great difficulty competing with his brother. His brother is four years his elder and was considered by his friends to be a "highly potent stud."

Giannis T. continues his account by telling me that he had the same difficulty competing with his brother in social settings, and he adds that this problem would also arise whenever he found himself faced with someone who, in one way or another, commanded his respect.

The patient, who is a very intelligent man, is unable to work in a consistent and effective manner, despite possessing a clear understanding of whatever task he needs to perform. He says that he has a tendency to suddenly fall into erotic reveries, even during working hours, and that he is often obliged to masturbate to clear his mind so that he can work more effectively and feel steady.

Giannis T. is a lawyer. He does not much care for his profession. He wanted, he says, to study literature and philosophy, but his father, knowing that his son had no interest in commerce, wanted to make an architect of him, in the belief that that profession would be more lucrative than the humanities. Lacking even the slightest affinity for that profession, the patient pleaded with his father to allow him to pursue the studies of his choice, but his father refused to give his consent. After several family scenes, the father proposed a compromise: he would allow his son to study law instead of architecture. In the end, Giannis T. accepted this compromise and did reasonably well until his third year, but had great difficulty completing his studies. He finally managed to obtain his degree, but only after repeating his final year twice.

In the meantime, his brother—who was four years older than the patient and had studied business—joined their father's business and began to lead an increasingly independent life. Giannis, by contrast, joined a prominent attorney's firm after graduating. Nonetheless, he remained highly dependent on his father, both psychologically and financially, because although he was a conscientious worker, he lacked initiative and his work left much to be desired. He always approached his work as though it were a great chore, and most of the time followed the instructions of the prominent lawyer, upon whom he was entirely dependent, despite how much this situation distressed him.

Giannis T. consoled himself by occupying himself with literature and philosophy. In this way, he found compensation for the painful feelings of inferiority he experienced when he compared himself to his father, his brother, his employer, and to anyone else who embodied a paternal type. He sought the company of intellectuals and artists, amongst whom he distinguished himself as a dialectician, showing brilliant intellectual capacities, especially in discussions of philosophy and aesthetics. (Later, in the course of the analysis, this talent as a dialectician was mobilized in the service of his resistances, leading to a prolongation of the treatment.)

After having spoken about his premature ejaculation, his inability to have erections with women who were not prostitutes or members of the lower classes, and his masturbation and feelings of inferiority, G. T. explained to me that he had tried, for quite some time, yet unsuccessfully, to cure himself through self-analysis, on the basis of the knowledge that he had gleaned from reading Freud. Then, attempting to be as precise as possible, he proceeded to describe some of his other symptoms, which he himself considered to be obsessional.

According to him, he felt a compulsive need to utter certain words. One of these words was the word "γαμόσταυρος" [*gamostauros*], which is a word composed of the verb "γαμῶ" [*gamō*], which, in Modern Greek, means "to fuck," and the word "σταυρός" [*stauros*], which means "cross"; the compound word "γαμόσταυρος" thus means "cross-fucker" or "he who fucks the cross." In Greece, this term is both an insult and blasphemous. At first, the patient would speak this word (in his head or whispered, and sometimes, when he was alone, aloud) in the nominative case, independently of any other word.

Later, he began to utter another word in the same manner, which, like the first word, he used for some time on its own in the nominative case. This was the word "πoύστης" [*poustēs*], which means "faggot." To this word, he later added the word "σκύλος" [*skylos*], meaning "dog," to create a second compound word, "σκυλοπούστης" [*skylopoustis*], which means "dog-faggot." Still later, he began to follow the first compound word with the second, and, by adding his own name, Giannis, to the two others, he would say these three words, one after the other, in the following order: "cross-fucker—dog-faggot—Giannis." From that time on, he stopped speaking these three words in the nominative and replaced that case by the vocative, meaning that he was directly addressing himself by these names, repeating them over and over again, and always in the same order.

Each time that someone mentioned either an illness or an accident that had befallen someone, in addition to shifting from his place, Giannis T. felt the imperious need to rub the thumb of his right hand repeatedly over the index finger of the same hand, because (although he wasn't superstitious overall) he had the feeling that if he didn't do this, either the person in question, or someone dear to him, might die.

Giannis T. also feels the need to wash his hands very frequently, even when his hands are perfectly clean.

He emphasizes that the images, or the erotic daydreams, that appear in his mind can neither be dispelled nor overcome effectively unless he masturbates.

Giannis T. distinguished between two varieties of masturbation: more-or-less impulsive masturbation, which was not accompanied by fantasies, and the type of masturbation he called "organized," which was by far the most frequent sort, and the most satisfying, and which was always accompanied by various erotic themes. At times, he said, these themes came into his mind on their own, and at other times, he would arrange them in his mind during the masturbatory act.

The patient also spoke to me about a tendency that he had of turning to other things at the very moment he was supposed to begin a professional task, or at the moment when he was supposed to finish one. He also has a tendency to ruminate endlessly on all sorts of ideas, trying to make them fit into philosophical frameworks or systems.

What I have just presented is more or less the condensed content of the three consultations that preceded the beginning of treatment.

Let us add, moreover, that the mother of Giannis T. died of pneumonia. The patient adds that, starting a few years after his mother's death, and up until the age of 14 or 15, he had a phobia of tuberculosis and would occasionally expectorate in order to check for blood in his sputum.

* * *

During the first four or five weeks of the treatment, the patient tended to bring material that had been deliberately arranged beforehand in spite of the fundamental rule, of which I ceaselessly reminded him. Gradually, however, once he came to better understand that this was just another form of resistance, this tendency diminished greatly, although it only completely disappeared several months later, along with his stubborn attempts at transforming his analysis into a scientific discussion, or into a discourse on art, philosophy and literature, in spite of my refusal to engage with him on these topics.

I shall now provide a few interesting elements that I have drawn from the material produced throughout the length of this treatment, selecting essential elements from amongst a great many others that I shall omit, in the interest of economy, whenever such omissions will not hamper the understanding of the case and of this paper. Otherwise, in order to describe all of the analytic work accomplished during this treatment, which lasted for over three years, I should have to write a very thick book on this case.

* * *

Following the death of the patient's mother, the older brother, who, up to that time, had attended primary school as a day student, was placed in a private academy, whilst a French governess was engaged for Giannis T. The father decided to keep him at home on account of his then-delicate constitution. Little Giannis, who had adored his mother, mourned her loss for a long time. Then, he redirected his love, not towards his governess, although she was very good to him, but towards a young chambermaid, who had entered the paternal household aged 19, about a year before his mother's death.

The patient reports that he had masturbated for the first time a short time before his mother's death, but I was able to ascertain that he had already been touching himself and engaging in masturbatory rubbing long before her death. He even remembers that a maid they used to have at the house, when he was five or six years old, told him that if he were to continue to touch his genitals, she would tell his father and that his father would cut them off, because this was a very great sin. Nonetheless, the patient did not stop playing with his genitals, and later on he would masturbate and experience great pleasure doing so, despite a feeling of guilt that persisted well past his adolescence.

This feeling later intensified when, one day, two years after his mother's death, the young servant girl whom the patient loved took advantage of the governess' day off and, using the pretext of playing with him, showed him her breasts and genitals, telling the young boy to touch them, while she manually stimulated his penis. From that time on, this young servant girl, whose name was Maria, would regularly come to "play" once a week (every Thursday) with young Giannis while the governess was out. She would masturbate him herself, and also would ask him to masturbate her, or to rub his penis on her clitoris and her labia, telling him that when he masturbated with a woman it was still sinful, but that the act was no longer deleterious to one's health, whereas by masturbating alone, one risked tuberculosis, imbecility, or madness. She further added that the sin of "playing" with a woman like this was much more easily forgiven than the sin of solitary pleasure, even by simply saying prayers, and that whenever he desired gratifications of this sort, he either had to wait until Thursday or, on other days of the week, find a way of meeting her in the storage room or in the attic. Maria ordered him to not say anything to his father, his brother, or his governess, and she continued to come play with him. Giannis wanted to meet her on the other days of the week, but he was too afraid of being found out by the governess, and he only very rarely saw Maria outside of the governess' days off, until the governess left the household for good, when he was nearly 12.

Besides mutual masturbation, Maria would also give him her nipples to suck, and would encourage him to rub his penis on her breasts. It was while doing this that he had his first ejaculation, a short while after the governess' departure, and about one year before entering the private academy (up to this time, he had been schooled by private tutors at home). From that time onwards, and despite the young servant girl's exhortations not to masturbate alone, he increasingly indulged in onanism, despite his more frequent relations with her.

Besides an increase in physiological pleasure, the ability to ejaculate gave Giannis two other contradictory feelings: on one hand, the pleasure of being capable of doing what his brother[2] and other adult men did, and, on the other hand, anxiety at the idea that by releasing his sperm, he might fall victim to dangerous or harmful consequences.

By this time, Giannis already knew a number of things about intercourse, but it was this young servant girl who, besides introducing him to the caresses of lovemaking, also revealed to him all of the details of normal coitus and impregnation. She also explained to him what virginity meant and told him that it was forbidden by both religion and the law to deflower virgins before a certain age or get them pregnant outside of marriage. But she explained to him that didn't mean that intercourse wasn't possible, and that young girls could do it, but in another way. So, Giannis, who already knew about the existence of anal intercourse from his brother, and who had imagined, during his infantile investigations, the theory of penile penetration of the anus and childbirth via the same route, asked her if she meant anal intercourse. Maria took on a mysterious air and refused to reply. Giannis got angry and threatened to break off their relations. So, the young servant girl replied in the affirmative, and told him that indeed, men could penetrate young girls' anuses and ejaculate there, without the risk of young girls or women becoming pregnant this way.

Giannis then asked her to allow him to penetrate her anally. Maria replied that anal intercourse was an even greater sin than the others, because it was an unnatural act, and she told him not to insist any further. Moreover, she told him, it is harder to penetrate the anus than the vagina, because of the tightness of the orifice, and she added: "You are too small to have the strength to penetrate me from that end." The patient vehemently insisted and begged her to let him try, especially since her last sentence had wounded him in his pride, but the young servant girl would hear nothing of it. Giannis persisted in his entreaties, and in the end, Maria, in exasperation, told him that she couldn't allow him to do it because there was another person who was already in the habit of doing this to her.

Stunned and profoundly upset by this revelation, the patient did not insist any further that day. The next day, the young boy, consumed by jealousy, asked the young servant girl again who it was that was doing it to her, but the young girl stubbornly refused to reveal the man's name. Giannis continued to beg, and, in the end, Maria offered a compromise: if he would kindly stop tormenting her with the question, as a reward, she would let him penetrate her. The patient accepted immediately. He had a good erection and made efforts to succeed, but they remained fruitless because of a minor accident that occurred at the culmination of his attempt. Giannis had a slight phimosis and, during his attempts to penetrate her, his foreskin tore slightly and began to bleed a bit. At the same time, he withdrew his penis just as he hoped to penetrate her and ejaculated. Frightened, Giannis did not repeat his attempt on that day. The chambermaid examined his penis and tried to calm him. Then, laughing, she told him that he had just lost his virginity and that he was now going to become a full-grown little man. But the patient, disturbed at the sight of blood, could not overcome his fright. So, the young servant girl, seeing his anxiety, said to him: "I was perhaps wrong to believe that you were going to become a little man . . . and that you would do what the other man does to me, because now you're acting like a little boy."

Two or three days afterwards, Giannis, having recovered from his fright, made a number of attempts on several occasions at inserting his penis into the young servant girl's anus but, each time, he ejaculated without achieving penetration. Marie's utterance, "I thought you'd do what the other man does to me; instead, you're acting like a little boy" was tormenting him like a burn. In the throes of disappointment, and feeling inferior to that unknown "other," he once again demanded that she tell him who that man was, but the young servant girl began to laugh and, as always, stubbornly refused to reveal the name to him. So, the young boy got angry and slapped her. Maria began to cry, but Giannis gave her another slap and threatened to tell his father everything. Thereupon, the young girl, seized with terror, promised to tell him her secret immediately, if the patient accepted to swear with a kiss on the little cross that she wore hanging against her chest, not to tell his father, his brother, or anyone else, and pulling the cross out from between her breasts, held it out to him. He swore upon the cross by kissing it, and the young maid entrusted him with her secret: "It's your father . . ." she said, and left the room, hiding her face in her apron.

Giannis T. tells me that he remained standing there, in shock. He had no further relations with the young servant girl and took quite some time to recover from the exceedingly and triply painful impression that Maria's revelation had made upon him. He analyses this triply painful impression. First of all, he had the feeling that his father was greatly superior to him, since he was capable of doing what he could not do. Secondly, that his father was morally inferior to what he had theretofore believed, since he also indulged in "unnatural" things. And thirdly, that his father was an enemy, since he came between him and the young servant girl. He, whom his son adored, had now become an enemy, but an enemy whom Giannis had to obey . . .

From that day on, the young boy broke off all intimacy with Maria. The young servant girl once attempted to make amends, telling him that he, Giannis, was the one she loved, but she accepted his father's propositions because she needed money, as he had promised her to double her wages if she accepted to have relations with him from time to time. She added that the father was a notorious womanizer, and that she had learned from the chauffeur's indiscretions that he had had a number of mistresses, as well as a *garçonnière* where he would take women with whom he was having relations, and so on and so forth. She also told him that she engaged in this method of intercourse in order to maintain her virginity intact, lest she be unable to marry later.

Despite his pain, Giannis felt very tempted to surprise his father with the maid, and having learnt that their relations generally took place at home in his father's office after the afternoon siesta when the chambermaid would bring him his coffee, he began to track Maria's movements and, one day, through the keyhole of the door leading from the parlor to the office, he saw his father having anal intercourse with the young servant girl.

Giannis T. tells me that never in his life would he forget the deeply disturbing impression made on him by, on one hand, the proportions of the paternal penis, and, on the other, the sex act itself, which he observed through to its end. It was a scene that he experienced as arousing yet terrifyingly violent—it was almost like a massacre, he says, especially since the young chambermaid was wincing in pain during the intromission and was making visible efforts, by biting her lips, not to cry out. And while Maria seemed to him like a torture victim, his father, standing behind her as he performed the rhythmic thrusting of intercourse as though he were possessed by mania, appeared to him like a monstrous and ferociously lustful large dog.

Later on, this scene would provide the material for certain sadomasochistic fantasies my patient had, but it also served as a screen-memory to prevent the recollection of other events of infantile life. This scene, says Giannis T., had unsettled him to an unimaginable degree. Yet, despite the anxiety and the deep sense of inferiority it instilled in him, its memory always set him ablaze, he said, as though it were an extremely arousing thing, and it awoke within him the desire to see it again. My patient succeeded in catching his father with the chambermaid on two or three other occasions before he left for the private academy, where he continued to masturbate to the recollection of Maria's image, amongst other images.

From that time on, Giannis' feelings towards his father changed. He regarded him with distrust and coldness, but this was mixed, he said, with an even greater admiration than before. The love he felt for him disappeared, while at the same time, his memory of his mother became even more sacred. And yet, my patient added, objectively his father's attitude towards him had not changed in the slightest. As always, he was authoritarian but benevolent, and he greatly loved both of his sons in his own way.

My patient finished his private school education at the age of 17. He had his first relations with a woman other than Maria at the age of 18. This was with a prostitute. Since that time, he has never stopped frequenting brothels but has always ejaculated prematurely. During his vacations and his travels, and during his military service, he also had relations with servant girls and workingwomen, all of which ended identically in premature ejaculations.

My patient's relationship with his brother, whom he esteemed greatly, had always remained, on the surface, very friendly. But, in reality, silent resentment against him filled Giannis' heart. This resentment and animosity were followed by remorse and feelings of guilt due to the benevolence his brother showed towards him, and the kindnesses through which the elder brother showed his affection for the younger. Moreover, Giannis' brother, from the time he entered University at the age of 18, wanted to make his younger brother his friend. But my patient, who was always intimidated and awkward in his brother's presence, could neither reciprocate nor enjoy his friendship. He always felt inferior in his brother's company, especially when women or young ladies were present, and he avoided any occasion that might put him in contact with his brother's girlfriends, especially because his brother had a lot of success with the opposite sex.

During the first months of his treatment, the patient readily accepted everything I told him about his father and his mother, he but displayed great difficulty taking in anything I told him about his reactions to me within the analytic situation.

I explained to him that even those elements of my interpretations that he accepted, and which were directly related to his feelings towards his parents, were in large part only accepted intellectually, artificially, without any emotional resonance, and were not the result of any true understanding. I added that, often, when he reacted in this way (i.e., officially and unilaterally accepting interpretations concerning his parents while rejecting the others), he was doing so in order to please me and to be at peace with me, instead of truly taking those interpretations in. By doing this, he was hiding his animosity towards me and was fleeing every possibility of seeing his repressed aggression resurface, in order to avoid the profound anxiety that his fear of castration caused him.

Characteristically, for quite some time, the patient would forget most of his dreams. And, all the while telling me that he wanted to help me in my analytic work, he would barricade himself more and more behind his resistances. We nonetheless continued our work without making any concession to his neurosis, and gradually we exited that phase by relentlessly attacking the resistances.

At last, the patient began to better understand his reactions and the manifestations of his transference, and insofar as he understood them better, he was able to proceed, albeit slowly, yet definitely, towards new phases that were increasingly rich in affective reactions, and which enabled a deeper elaboration of the contents of the neurosis through the reviviscence of various constitutive elements of his unconscious organization.

* * *

In the case of Giannis T., it is possible to distinguish between two groups of symptoms which appear in the same layer of the psyche and manifest simultaneously: the disturbances of sexual function and the obsessional symptoms.

As regards the former group, during the treatment of Jean T. and in other analogous cases, I have frequently had the opportunity of remarking upon the accuracy of observation, the depth of understanding, and the finesse of the psychoanalytic explanation by which the great student of Freud, Karl Abraham, treats the subject of premature ejaculation in his admirable work on this sexual disorder written in 1917. The lessons in this paper were of great help to me in the case of Giannis T., not only in understanding the nature of the disorder, but also in helping my patient be rid of it.

In chapter II of this paper, Abraham says:

> We may say that premature ejaculation occurs in those men who are burdened with strong—partly unconscious, partly conscious—resistances against activities of a specifically masculine character.
>
> The neurotic type who is without energy usually expresses a conscious antipathy towards exercising any activity in sexual matters; he even has an open desire to assume the female role. One of my patients liked to play the part of the succubus, and gave as a reason for this that if he paid a girl he did not want to have to exert himself as well—that she ought to "work" for her money. Naturally, neurotic persons with this degree of displeasure in movement are not favourable subjects for medical treatment, particularly if they consciously defend their abnormality. Their chief desire is to attain sexual gratification without taking any active part in it. . . .
>
> The inertness and passivity exhibited by these neurotics is, however, a reactive manifestation. It can be found that such an attitude has taken the place of a too forcible sadistic impulse. The tendency to be quarrelsome, to have fits of anger, and to commit violent acts, is extraordinarily marked in such people, in so far as it is not paralyzed by another character-trait which distinguishes them—namely, cowardice. Excessive irascibility and a paralysis of the normal male pleasure in attack are found here in close proximity. The frequent juxtaposition of excessive ambition and severe resistance against work is also met with in this group of neurotic persons. . . .
>
> If we allow ourselves to be guided by the free associations of the patients, we learn that originally their libido was not lacking in a sadistic

> component. Psycho-analysis teaches us that in most of the cases, besides the unmanly and passive or precipitate and over-active attitude, there exists in the unconscious an aggressive and cruel attitude towards the feminine. In their dreams and in other products of phantasy these patients often produce the idea of killing the woman by copulating with her. In these phantasies the penis is the sadistic weapon. . . .
>
> The associations of the patient indicate in addition, moreover, that in their unconscious ejaculatio præcox signifies the extreme opposite of killing.[3]

I cite these passages in order to add that, having identified a number of similarities in the case of Giannis T., I was able to draw therapeutic benefit from them, of course not by giving my patient theoretical lectures, but by fruitfully using the lessons contained in Abraham's work in my analytic interpretations of the manifest and latent material my patient gave me regarding his premature ejaculations.

I shall add that having asked the patient whether he had episodes of urinary incontinence during his youth, he replied that he had continued to wet the bed from time to time up to the age of five or six. This declaration was followed by several memories illustrating this fact.

A few of the analytic interpretations I made regarding the second group of symptoms will be presented later on in this paper.

Here, I must explain myself on several points.

On the basis of certain dream elements, on a series of associations, and on certain of my patient's fantasies, I had tried to show him the accuracy of my opinion, according to which his discovery that the chambermaid Maria was having relations with his father, while it was a traumatic element (the patient attributed the genesis of his neurosis solely to that episode), was neither the primary nor the sole cause of his difficulties. I had added that, although that episode played an important role in the formation and basic elements of the neurosis, I had the impression that there were other events in the patient's life that had played a traumatic role.

Indeed, taking into account, on one hand, the material supplied by my patient and his affective reactions, and, on the other hand, drawing on the magnificent clinical and theoretical works of Freud, as well as on my own therapeutic experience, I had the impression that the primal scene was still escaping us, as well as a number of elements that doubtlessly had that scene at their core.

The Oedipal manifestations as well as the reactions emanating from the regression of the libido to the pregenital stages were clearly visible in his relations with me, and he experienced anxiety each time that, as a result of my interpretations, he was faced with their meaning within both his neurosis and the analytic situation.

A sentence, spoken one day by Giannis T., gave me the opportunity to help him see more clearly certain aspects of his reactions, not only to his father and his mother and me, but also towards himself, which had theretofore completely escaped him.

This was the sentence: "Mr. Embiricos, it seems that you want to spoil my transference."

I seized this opportunity to explain to him that not only did he have a great deal of anxiety about accepting his aggression towards his father and towards me, a great deal of difficulty stepping outside of his narcissism and ceasing his passive attitude to accept rivalry with his father and his analyst to win for himself the mother and the woman, but that he also feared losing the possibility of obtaining passive feminine gratification through his identification with his mother.

The worry that I might spoil the transference by my interpretations represented not only his fear of losing me, if he used his penis in a complete and virile way by being in competition with me for women—meaning accepting rivalry with his father—but also, the worry, and the sentence that expressed it ("you want to spoil my transference"), made manifest the anxiety he experienced each time that he had to accept and take on an active orientation towards women (the mother) by ceasing his unconscious attempts at being, as he wished to be, the object of his analyst's libido, the object of the maternal and paternal libido, or the object of his own libido in a narcissistic manner. Worrying that I might spoil the transference was another expression of his desire to maintain a passive attitude within the analysis, as in eros, with the goal of attaining urethral, passive orgasm (premature ejaculation) as when he urinated, and to completely do away with the need of directing his erect penis, penetrating a woman, and actively releasing his sperm within the vagina via the rhythmical movements of coitus. There was such multiplicity of meaning in this sentence that it also allowed me to show my patient how anal erotism also played a role in the etiology of his premature ejaculations (the patient sometimes had anal spasms while ejaculating). It also displayed his fear of independence, because of his desire to retain my erect penis inside of him (prolonged ruminations on various ideas, interminable ruminations on my interpretations, a tendency to transform them into verbal formulas stripped of their true meaning). Finally, this phase, and the color of the affect with which it was charged, allowed us to see the resentment my patient harbored towards me because of the fact that I didn't "go along with" his passive desires and demands, which were unconscious, and which had taken the place of his repressed aggression.

* * *

As I stated earlier, I had the impression that behind the dramatic episode of the discovery of the chambermaid's relations with his father, other experiences were hiding, and that behind that event from the first years of G. T.'s adolescence, other traumatic elements lay hidden beneath the more recent layers which formed, from within the deepest strata of his unconscious, the true source of his neurosis.

I shared this opinion with my patient and drew his attention to the fact that, although he often spoke to me about his relations with the chambermaid and the event that put an end to these relations, he never, or almost never, spoke to me about any earlier events.

The patient stated that he did not believe that I was right, and he told me that his childhood, besides his fragile health and the pain he experienced at losing his mother, had been without turmoil.

I reminded him of the threats of castration his maid had made when she surprised him playing with his penis, of his urinary incontinence which continued until the age of six, of his father's strictness, of his feelings of guilt after masturbating, and I added that even his fragile health should very probably also be seen as a psychic reaction. But G. T. maintained his point of view.

Yet a dream he had after the end of the first year of analysis shook his sense of certainty. Here is that dream:

> The patient finds himself between two acts in the foyer of a theater with an unknown lady. The lady asks him for a cigarette. He takes out his cigarette case, but instead of offering her a cigarette, he puts it in her mouth. Just as the cigarette is about to touch the lady's lips, a man wearing a cap with a big pipe in his mouth approaches and takes the cigarette from his hands. The patient turns to "tell him off" but remains silent and motionless for a few moments, unable to express his anger, and then the three of them leave together.

Associations: Giannis T. very much likes the theater. His father did not allow him to smoke in front of him until after his military service. He did not smoke much until his second year in University, but at that time he began to smoke heavily. The lady does not remind him of anyone, he says at first, but then, changing his mind, he adds: "Maybe she resembles my mother a little bit." The gesture of putting the cigarette in the woman's mouth reminds him that he sometimes used to ask women to suck his penis. Ejaculation would then occur almost immediately, as during his attempts at coitus. As a child, he used to love the adventures of Sherlock Holmes, and Sherlock Holmes himself, who was always able to catch the criminal and solve the most difficult problems through his powerful reasoning and his shrewd perspicacity.

Interpretation: After having seen one act (the loves and conflicts of others) on stage, he enters the foyer with his mother, in order to, at last, do what actors (lovers) do, instead of remaining a spectator (voyeur). He places a cigarette in his mother's mouth, displacement from below to above, the vagina in the place of the mouth, as though he were preparing to penetrate her. But this gesture has a double meaning. It also expresses the desire to receive pleasure from his mother's mouth, as mouth, meaning it expresses his desire to be fellated by her and to passively attain orgasm by the action of her lips and tongue, and identifying with her in a way that corresponds to the inversion of the oral pleasure he himself had as an infant sucking on his mother's nipples.

Here, I emphasized (reminding the patient of an interpretation I had made of prior associations) that he could not see a woman's vagina without anxiety, because the sight of the female genital always reactivated his fear of becoming castrated like a woman, because to him, women, due to their vagina, were both castrated beings and victims.

Now, I shall return to my interpretation. At the very moment he is preparing to perform this sex act with its double meaning, the analyst (Sherlock Holmes), father substitute, who discovers and sheds light on all the mysteries (repressed desires and anxieties) of his unconscious, arrives with his big penis (the big pipe, compared to his thin cigarette) and cuts off his penis. But the analyst in his dream doesn't just cut off his penis; he also cuts off his pleasure by triggering his rivalry through his interpretations and making him face the reality that he wants to flee through denial and avoidance of competition with his father.

It can therefore be said that in this scene, both the fear of castration and castration itself appear, because Sherlock Holmes takes the cigarette from him, but at the same time (following the expression of the patient's desire to have relations with his mother), it can be seen how the patient, by having himself castrated and avoiding expressing his anger towards me, seeks to obtain, in compensation for this great sacrifice, my love and my penis, meaning the privilege of staying by my side, like the mother. Thus, he does not attack me, but he causes himself to be attacked by me, and instead of leaving alone with his mother, the three of us leave together. The patient has himself castrated not only to punish himself, but also in order to obtain pleasure through me, as he did through his mother.

But there was another element in this dream that made an impression on me. The patient had said that he was located in the lobby of a theater *between two acts* and not at the *entr'acte*.[4] After having made the foregoing interpretation, I added another interpretation, which might have seemed a bit arbitrary, but which later revealed itself to be absolutely justified.

Thus, I said to my patient:

> When you told me your dream, you said you were with that lady in the foyer of a theater *between two acts* and not at the *entr'acte*. It might be possible that you were alluding to the fact that you were located not only between two acts of a play, but also between two *acts* that took place in your life, and which are, perhaps, the two acts that played the most important role in your psychic development. The first might be the anal sex *act* between your father and the chambermaid, which you observed, which upset you so greatly, and of which you have often spoken to me; and the other, a sex *act* that was similar or analogous, but earlier, and which you might have observed, too, and perhaps which upset you to the same degree, or even more, and whose conscious memory escapes you.

And I added:

> You speak French quite well, and you know that in French the word *foyer* also means *maison familiale* [the family home], *le chez soi* [one's own home]. It may therefore be said that you are alluding to two independent scenes, both of which took place in your own home, at your house, which had been the *theater* of these scenes, where you saw these two acts unfold, and the first of which, the earlier one, still escapes your memory today.

* * *

This interpretation made an impact on my patient that was so great that I momentarily thought that we were possibly going to see the memory of the primal scene—or of some other important event in our patient's life—rise up from infantile amnesia. But this would only occur later. We still had a long road to travel. Without becoming discouraged, I resigned myself to wait for the treatment to develop further.

The patient, after having heard this interpretation, said to me in an emotional tone: "I think that that interpretation, and especially what you added to it afterwards, is one of the most important and the most impressive I have yet heard from you . . ." and then he fell into a brief silence that lasted until the time I stood up, as the analytic hour had come to an end.

The next day, Giannis T. told me that during these few moments of silence, and then in the street, on his way home, as he thought about my interpretation, he had pronounced the compound words *cross-fucker* and *dog-faggot* followed by another name than his own, and he asked me to guess whose name he had put in the place of his own.

I remained silent, although I was tempted to say that he had undoubtedly used mine. The patient, piqued by my silence, told me: "I put your name in the place of my own, calling you the cross-fucker and the dog-faggot . . ."

The patient lapsed into silence. I continued not to speak and after one or two minutes, Giannis T. broke his silence to tell me that the famous silence of the analyst is sometimes like a humiliation for his patient . . .

At last, I began to speak.

You can imagine what interpretative use I made of everything that Giannis T. had told me since the start of that session. I regret that for reasons of space, in order to be able to incorporate more important things in this study, I am obliged to omit the interpretation I made at this moment, which was interesting and useful. I shall add, in any case, that my patient's reactions, which I have just described, showed that the prior day's interpretations were beginning to bear fruit as the patient was able to put my name instead of his following the two compound words he used obsessively, addressing them to a father substitute for the first time, in an attacking way, instead of addressing them to himself.

That same day, I asked my patient to give me new associations to his two compound words.

After a pause, Giannis T. told me that the word *cross-fucker* reminded him of the little cross that hung between Maria's breasts (the chambermaid) and upon which he had spilt his semen when he ejaculated for the first time. From that day on, the young servant girl would remove her cross each time he rubbed his penis on her breasts. This word also reminded him of the promise he had sworn on that same cross, when, in order to reveal to him the name of her other lover (who was Giannis' father), she had made him swear upon the cross, by making him kiss it, that he would never repeat to anyone else the secret she was about to tell him.

For quite some time, I believed that those two events had engendered the obsessional neologisms that my patient had been compulsively repeating for such a long time. And it was only later that I discovered that there had been yet another event.

Let us return to my patient's associations to the two compound words.

The word *dog-faggot* oriented Giannis T.'s thoughts to the time when he was in secondary school. At the age of 14, about a year after the end of his relations with the chambermaid, he became friendly with a classmate of the same age, who demonstrated a homosexually friendly, ardent attachment towards him. At first, this only manifested itself on the emotional level, but then it became openly homosexual. During this latter period, this boy wanted to have relations with Giannis, but my patient refused his friend's advances for a long time. But, one day (the day before school let out for the holidays), Giannis, who was still frequently secretly masturbating, gave in to his classmate's entreaties and allowed him to masturbate him, and he returned the favor, in the school toilets. When school began again after the vacation, that boy did not return to school. The schoolboys, and our patient among them, wondered why. Finally, a classmate told him that there was a rumor going around that the principal had learned that boy was a "faggot" and did not want him in the establishment any longer. Giannis said that he never figured out whether that rumor was true, or whether it was a malevolent lie, but he was personally very inclined to believe that it must have been true. In any case, this painfully affected Giannis, and for a long time he could not hear the word *faggot* without blushing and without thinking that others might suspect him, too, of being homosexual, even though, he added, he only liked women.

The word *faggot* also reminded my patient that one day, his father's chauffeur, upon seeing his father's hunting dog mounting another male dog, shouted in his presence: "Goddamn ass-fucker, have you no shame?" Giannis could not say what age he was exactly when this occurred, but he said it took place sometime before his mother's death. The same day, the patient asked his brother what the word "κωλομπαράς" [*kōlomparas*] meant, and his brother, laughing, answered that it meant "one who fucks asses." Giannis did not know what the verb *fuck* meant, and so he asked his brother what the meaning was, and his brother, putting the index finger of his right hand into the closed fist of his left hand, made a back-and-forth motion with his finger in and out of the fist, and said "to fuck" meant doing that with a man's "pee-pee" inside of a woman's "pee-pee."

Giannis T., who had already observed canine intercourse, and who had "an inkling," he said, that men might do the same to women, but because he believed that men and dogs alike penetrated the anus, felt surprised that a man or a dog could penetrate another orifice than the anus, and, later, when he paid closer attention, he realized that male dogs penetrated female dogs' vaginas and not their anuses.

Giannis' older brother, seeing his surprise, added: "Imbecile, don't you know that all men do it to women in the cunt?" That's how Giannis learned the vulgar word for the female organ. And Giannis' brother added: "Papa does it to Mama, too."

At that point, the patient sat up halfway on the couch and, turning towards me, said:

> You are right, now I see that well before my relations with the chambermaid, and well before the observation of her anal intercourse with my father, I was already overwhelmed by those things . . . Moreover, the verb "γαμῶ" (to fuck) forms part of the compound "γαμόσταυρος" (cross-fucker) . . . Doubtlessly, I associated that word with my father's sexual activity with my mother and, later on, with my own sexual activity with the chambermaid who wore the little cross on her chest. I remember now that when I was a child, and even after I had grown, and even to this day, every time I saw a male dog mounting a bitch in the street or in the countryside, I've had very intense heart palpitations, but I thought that it was only due to excitement, without sufficiently understanding that at the same time, there was anxiety causing those palpitations . . .

* * *

During the four or five weeks after that important session, Giannis T.'s tendency to compulsively repeat the compound words diminished in intensity and frequency without disappearing entirely, and he then brought me the following dream.

> I find myself in a large, somber garden with my father. He is remarried to a young blonde woman, and the three of us are walking together. My father tells me to go buy him some sandwiches. I go, but instead of buying sandwiches, I buy flowers from a young woman florist seated in a fantastical kiosk-car driven by an officer. When I return to my father, the garden seems brighter, less gloomy, and instead of my father's second wife, I see the young florist, to whom I present the flowers. The young lady asks me, "Are these flowers for me or for my husband?" I answer that the flowers are for her.

Giannis T. tells me that there was a continuation to this dream, but he no longer remembers it.

> Associations: The large, somber garden reminds Giannis T. of cemeteries. The patient then tells me that he feels very moved, because he just remembered something that happened when he visited his mother's tomb for the first time, along with his father and his brother. Looking at the cross on the tomb upon which they had just placed flowers, he thought he saw, for an instant, the image of his mother, crucified, dying in agony, while a Roman soldier pierced her side with a spear—and he fainted.

The patient's emotion prevented him from speaking for a few moments, and then he told me that he felt that this memory must be important for his treatment. He said that at the first Easter after his mother's death, he had prayed fervently that God resurrect his mother, as Christ had been resurrected. He added that he could now understand that perhaps the primary cause of his atheism was that God had not fulfilled that prayer.

Then, Giannis T. told me that about two years prior to his analysis, he had taken a young itinerant flower-seller aged 12 or 13 to a *maison de passe*, promising her a generous sum of money if she allowed him to have fun with her without causing her any harm—by which he meant that he intended to leave her virginity intact.

The little girl accepted. Once they'd arrived at the *maison de passe*, G. T. asked her to show him her genitals and, after having examined them closely (he said it was in order to learn what the difference was between a young girl's and an adult woman's genitals), he positioned her so as to attempt to penetrate her anally, but he ejaculated "*ante portas*." Giannis held the girl against himself and masturbated her. Then, he wanted to pleasure himself with her again, this time by rubbing his penis on the girl's labia and clitoris "while imagining that he was going to deflower her" but, at the first contact, he ejaculated almost immediately. The little girl, who was very excited, began to rub her clitoris all by herself until she attained orgasm, and the patient carefully observed the expression on her face and listened to her sighs and the exclamations of pleasure that escaped from her mouth, and he began to masturbate again.

This scene led Giannis to another association. One summer night, when he was 11 years old, during a heatwave, he could no longer sleep and walked barefoot to the open window to get a bit of air. Suddenly, he heard a bed creaking and barely-stifled moans from the adjacent bedroom, which belonged to his French governess—a sweet, kindly woman of about 35. He left the window, looked through the keyhole of the door that led from his room to hers, and saw his governess unclothed, masturbating on the bed. He saw everything, he said, up to the orgasm, which impressed him as much as the act itself.

From that time on, he remained on alert so that he would be able to catch his governess masturbating again. But he wasn't able to see her often, first of all because she didn't seem to caress herself very frequently, but also because of the darkness, when this would happen at night. So, he would restrict himself to listening to her sighs, while masturbating himself while the governess was doing the same. It was only when the Frenchwoman did it during the afternoon, during the siesta, which rarely happened, that he was able to see, and he observed with great avidity and lust, and always up to the end, the act by which his governess gave herself pleasure.

He would record the most minor details, the movement of the fingers on the genital organ when the governess was unclothed, the swooning expressions of pleasure that also felt worrisome to him, the muffled sighs, the little cries when she couldn't contain herself, up to the crest, up to the spasmodic jerks of the final culmination of pleasure, while he masturbated himself immediately after or during the observation, while great shivers of pleasure ran through his body, and he said he experienced a profoundly lascivious ecstasy, but which was also accompanied by anxiety and terrible heart palpitations.

Here, a brief silence followed this story. Then Giannis T. said to me that he was thinking about something regarding his mother, which had already come into his mind the day that he told me about the dogs, but that he wasn't able to tell me that day. Again, he lapsed into silence. Finally, the patient told me that about a year prior to his mother's death, he went into his mother's boudoir and saw her, lying on the couch, reading a book. Just as he entered, his mother, who was wearing a bathrobe, moved and a little Pekinese who belonged to her came out from between her legs, lifting up the bathrobe slightly, and jumped to the floor. Giannis' mother seemed a bit troubled, and she said to the little dog: "Bobby, aren't you ashamed of yourself, you tore my robe . . . You deserve a beating!"

And the patient continued:

> It is likely that the little dog was just sleeping between my mother's legs or at her feet, and that I had awoken him by entering, but I wondered whether before my arrival the Pekinese hadn't burrowed even higher, up to my mother's genitalia, and whether he hadn't been licking them, as I had often seen dogs do to one another, when I entered the room.
>
> I don't know what happened in my mother's boudoir, and I repeat that most probably nothing happened, but for a long time, I could not free my mind of that suspicion, and then another suspicion was added to it, namely that perhaps my mother would allow the Pekinese to penetrate her, and also my father's big hunting dog of whom she was also very fond. These sacrilegious thoughts came into my mind quite often, despite myself, in the form of fantasies, as you say, for a long time, even years after my mother's death. I felt intense anxiety each time I thought of such things, and I felt deep shame, accompanied by feelings of guilt, because I, her son, was capable of having such thoughts or conjuring up such images regarding

> my mother, who was not only a very beautiful woman, but also the personification of goodness, sweetness and refinement, and whom I adored.

Then the patient told me that after having discovered that his governess masturbated, he often wondered (with the same reactions of anxiety and guilt) whether his mother didn't also masturbate. And he said that he often wondered if his mother hadn't in fact died of pneumonia, but rather because of his father's brutal penetration, on one hand, but also because of her masturbation and what she was doing with the dogs, on the other.

And he continued:

> I must therefore emphasize that after what my brother had told me during our conversation about dogs, which ended with the sentence, "Papa does it to Mama, too," despite my attempts not to pin on my father such a violent and cruel activity in his secret relations (that is how I sometimes termed his sexual relations with my mother), each time that I thought about those relations, I imagined my father treating my mother in such a way as to cause her to suffer; his role must have been bestial, since he was doing the same thing as dogs did.

As the associations in this session did not leave me much time, I decided to delay interpreting the dream until the following day's session, and reminding my patient of the sentence that his mother said to the Pekinese ("Aren't you ashamed of yourself, you tore my robe . . . You deserve a beating"), I asked him the following question: "Do you remember ever having looked up your mother's skirts, or your maids' skirts, as a boy, and to have been punished for that?"

Very spontaneously, the patient replied:

> Yes, at the age of about four or five I looked up the skirts of a little girl who used to play with us while she was urinating in the garden, and I saw her little genital organ. At the time, I was a much more rambunctious child than I was later on. One of the following days, I wanted to see what my maid's genitals looked like, and I lifted up her skirt. The maid scolded me and threatened to tell my parents. Despite her threat, because I had seen nothing else under her skirts besides her panties, I tried again, repeating the same gesture, not on the maid, but on a young servant girl in our home. Because she resisted, I became aggressive and tore at her petticoat . . . Then the young servant girl became angry and told my mother, in front of my father, and she added, I believe, that I had scratched her thighs, which might have happened because of how persistent I was being. My father summoned me and gave me a good beating . . .

I seized upon this occasion to show Giannis T. that that scene, which had taken place a number of years before the scene in the boudoir, doubtlessly reminds him of his own desires to see and, more than likely, to touch not only the maids' genitals, but also his mother's, and that the sight of the genitals of the little girl urinating had caused him such anxiety because of the absence of a penis. And I added that when he wanted to see his maids' genitals, it was certainly for the pleasure of seeing those hidden parts, but also to investigate whether all women lacked a male organ or not, and to calm the anxiety caused by his suspicion they all lacked a penis. It was the sight of the little girl's genitals and other such realizations that were probably even older, that must have suggested to him the idea or the image of castration.

I also said to him that when his mother told the little dog, "Aren't you ashamed you tore my dress . . . You deserve a beating!" he associated the tearing of the dress with the tearing of the maternal genitals, which he attributed to his father's activities, who had a bigger penis than his small child's penis. He had, perhaps, already seen either the father's penis or the penis of another adult man, and certainly his brother's penis, who was four years older than him . . .

And I added that he was already afraid at that point, as later, to give in to his own desires: if he saw, if he touched, if he took pleasure in his mother's genitals, as well as all of its hidden charms, he would deserve not only to be beaten, but to be castrated by his father, and would become like the little girl, a castrated being, like his mother and other women, especially since he had already been beaten, at the age of four, by that same father (that he identified with dogs) for having wanted to concern himself with sexual things.

I also told Giannis T. that already at that point, as later, he wanted to take the place of the dog in what he suspected it did to his mother (cunnilingus, coitus), acts that he wanted to perform himself, but that whether or not his mother had allowed herself to be licked by the dogs, he could not accept as his own the desires that he projected onto her.

As he did nearly each time that an interpretation made a significant impression on him, this time, too, the patient sat up halfway and looked at me.

"I believe," he said, "that now I understand not only what you have just said to me, but also a whole lot of similar things that you have interpreted to me, and that up to now, I only understood imperfectly."

The mere sight of women's genitals caused him anxiety, but at the same time, he said, he desired to look at them. He now had a much better understanding of his voyeurism.

He had always been very voyeuristic. He enjoyed watching other peoples' sexual relations, wherever he could, in hotels, in *maisons de passe*, as well as intercourse between animals.

* * *

The next day, I interpreted the dream whose manifest content took place in a garden, and in which he sees his father with a woman whom he has remarried, and this woman is later replaced by the flower girl he had bought flowers from and he gave this girl those flowers after she had taken the place of his father's second wife in the dream (see above).

Before interpreting, I asked my patient what associations he had to the sandwiches he mentioned in the dream, as well as the automobile kiosk, and the young blonde woman at the start of the dream.

Giannis T. replied that he always takes sandwiches with him whenever he takes a trip somewhere. Then, he told me that he had heard it said that when a man sleeps with two women and that he makes love between them, that is called a "sandwich," and also when two men sleep with a woman at the same time, and they penetrate her simultaneously vaginally and anally, that is also called a "sandwich," and he added that although he had always wanted to sleep with two women at the same time, he hadn't yet done so.

The fantastic automobile-kiosk reminds him of the little wagon-shops drawn by horses that one sees in the provinces, belonging to merchants who sell fabrics and small feminine items to peasant women and village girls. Then the patient adds: "This automobile-kiosk in the dream also reminds me, on one hand, of the flower-covered cars that parade during flower festivals, and on the other hand, of funeral hearses."

The young blonde woman at the start of the dream reminds my patient of Maria, the chambermaid, who was blonde, and whom the woman in the dream rather resembled. Later, when Maria left his father's household, she married a vegetable seller.

Interpretation of the dream: The patient's father is remarried in the dream, he is walking with his new wife and his son in a large, somber garden which my patient finds reminiscent of cemeteries. This same man's bestial brutality (dogs, dog's coitus, father's coitus with mother) was held by my patient to have been the main reason for his mother's death. This garden is therefore the cemetery where his sweet and good mother was buried, having been his father's victim: the cemetery where the little boy fainted, the day when he visited his mother's tomb for the first time, upon which he laid flowers, after having believed he'd seen his mother crucified and pierced like Christ by the spear of a Roman soldier (Roman soldier piercing with his spear: father who castrates and kills using his phallus, a cross-fucker). The father, who is very much a womanizer in reality, takes as many women as he can. In the dream, he takes the young blonde woman who reminds my patient of Maria, the chambermaid with whom he sexually amused himself until he discovered that his father was having relations with her—"unnatural" relations (as the chambermaid used to say), bestial relations. The father is taking this young woman (Maria) from him in the dream, as he had done in reality, and just as he had already deprived the son of his beloved mother—the mother who had been subjected to the father's intercourse in a way that tortured and victimized her, not only by penetrating her anally, but also from the front, after having cut off her penis; for the patient had believed that all women possessed a penis before he had discovered the difference between the sexes.

The patient's father orders him to go buy sandwiches and thereby to distance himself. Why should he have to distance himself? So that the father can be alone with the young blonde lady, Maria, so that he can have relations with her.

I explained that here, there is another meaning. When G. T. distances himself on his father's orders, he is also expressing the opposite desire to see his father distance himself, the desire of eliminating him and taking his place beside the blonde, which he cannot yet do in dream. G. T. obeys at the cost of his own humiliation, because he is sent off to do the type of shopping that is more commonly done by women.

Moreover, I explained to him, that he sees two women in this dream—the two women whom he had most loved in his childhood: the florist-mother (his mother used to love flowers) and the young blonde woman, his father's second wife at the start of the dream, who is the chambermaid Maria. He finds himself between these two women, like the men in one of his associations who lie between two women, making love in a "sandwich" with both at the same time. And I add that a part of him (following his identification with the mother-victim and his inability to become independent, first affectively and then socially, from his father) would like to be able to, in the opposite direction, lie between two men—his father and his brother or me, or between a phallic woman, with the penis of one in his anus (spasms in the anus during his premature ejaculations) and the penis of the other in a hypothetical vagina (orifice remaining in place of his severed penis). Then, he would feel full and complete, in compensation for the abdication of his penis, meaning in compensation for his castration (inability to penetrate women, premature ejaculations outside of the vagina, masturbation with fantasies representing him often passively reaching orgasm with women or young girls who actively give him pleasure, frequenting prostitutes from whom he purchases sexual satisfactions, inability to work fruitfully as a lawyer, financial dependence on his father, and professional dependence on his employer).

But, I said, pursuing my interpretation, we can see that you have made an important step forward in this dream. Instead of bringing back sandwiches, you disobeyed your father and brought back flowers that you offered to your father's second wife in the dream, the blonde woman who becomes the florist that you had bought those flowers from a few minutes earlier, instead of delivering them to your father, telling her that those flowers are for her. Despite this step forward, however, there are other steps that you are not yet ready to take. You are too scared of your father, you don't make him take his distance, you stay there, and you watch him. You are afraid that, on one hand, if you show your sexual interest in your mother-florist, she will die, and on the other hand, that you might become a sadistic brute, a copulating dog, a cross-fucker—meaning a fucker-crucifier of sweet and good women, a rival to your father, and that you will therefore be castrated by him. So, you simultaneously fear losing what you hope to obtain from him by remaining well-behaved, harmless, a premature ejaculator, passively orgasming, without either penetrating—or killing—the woman.

I once again reminded my patient that after his return from purchasing the flowers, the place of the young blonde woman (Maria) was taken by the florist (mother). I seize upon this opportunity to remind him that the chambermaid had always been a mother substitute, and I add that the fact that she takes Maria's place beside the father in the dream shows us that the patient wants her to take this place beside him. But at the same time, this scene indicates that he is still afraid of accepting that she might return (be resurrected) for him, because that would signify that he has accepted rivalry with his father, that he sees her once again as his father's wife, which enables him to be close to her in a safe way, a way that is allowed by his father, his own super-ego, and society as a whole.

I remind him, too, that he had said that upon returning with the flowers, he found the garden cheerier and less somber than at the start of the dream, and I explain to him:

> You are afraid, in the dream, that if you push your gallantry any further, you'll once again transform the garden, which has become a garden of love, into a garden of death (cemetery), that the mother-florist will die, and that you yourself will lose your life, in the event that you accept eliminating-killing your father.

Here, I asked G. T. whether in the meantime he had been able to remember the final scene of this dream, and as the patient replied in the negative, I continued:

> One might well wonder whether, perhaps, in the final scene that you say you forgot, you took one more step forward. In this case, you might object that the last part of my interpretation is not correct. In reply, I will say that the fact that you have forgotten this scene justifies the final part of my interpretation.

And I ended by explaining to G. T. the meaning of the fantastic car-kiosk, in which the florist is seated at the point where he purchases the flowers. This car-kiosk is the opposite of the hearse; it is a nuptial automobile, the type of automobile one sees at flower festivals, an automobile of virginal joy, so long as he does not consummate the sex act with the florist. Were said consummation to occur, he fears that the car would be transformed into a hearse, like the one that bore his mother to the cemetery!

And, I concluded, G. T. has made an important step forward by disobeying his father and by giving the flowers to the florist, but he is afraid of making the final gesture both of taking the mother as the father does, but also of castrating the father; he stands there looking at the young florist and forgets the final scene of this extremely important dream.

* * *

Following the interpretation of that dream and the analysis of the highly interesting associations the patient made that day, I noticed increased progress and noticeably more rapid improvement.

One of the signs of the improvement underway was that the compulsive compound words *cross-fucker* and *dog-faggot* gradually disappeared. Another sign was an improvement in the patient's ability to compete with the brother and the attorney who was his employer. Nonetheless, G. T. continued to frequent brothels and to always ejaculate prematurely. He also continued to masturbate.

This state of affairs lasted for nearly a year. I still had the idea that the primal scene was yet eluding me. Despite the profusion of highly useful elements from the patient's puberty, adolescence and young adulthood, and which I was able to use effectively, I still felt that the kernel constituting the main source of this neurosis remained buried in the deepest layers of the unconscious. Moreover, despite the progress made, the premature ejaculations continued! And the patient still restricted himself to relations with purchasable women.

Our patient's libido had not yet become disengaged from its infantile cathexes. His conflict with his father had not yet been completely accepted. The dreams showed this, and the more his aggression, although camouflaged, towards his father and me increased, the more his fear of castration grew. I recognized this at every instance where he had to face such rivalry, particularly since it was necessary, in order to conquer the father within him, to overcome his dependency on him and on the analyst.

This fear, as well as the pregenital fixations, continued to impede the libido's evolution towards adult amorous activity and hindered the patient in his journey from narcissism to object choice.

But we continued our analytic work patiently, and lo and behold, one day my patient brought me the following important dream:

> The patient is on the terrace of a villa, near the seaside, with a well-known American cinema actress who is wearing a beautiful white dress. It is a lovely summer night, and he is caressing the young woman's breasts, while he listens to the distant murmur of the tide. He has an erection, and he wants to have intercourse with her. He wants to ask her to give herself to him, but he is hesitating. Then, he makes up his mind, he leans in and kisses her on the mouth, but he has the feeling that something is flowing out from his lips onto hers and he immediately interrupts the kiss. At the same time, the actress faints and slips from his arms onto the paving stones. Then, G. T. notices that there are bloodstains on the white dress,

on his sweater, and that blood is still flowing out of the young woman's lips. G. T. wants to lift her up to carry her into her bedroom, but he cannot, because of the incredible weight of the young woman's body, and he awakens in a state of anxiety.

Associations: The patient had gone to the cinema with a friend two or three days prior to this dream, and he saw a film whose heroine was a Hollywood star, whom G. T. finds to be very attractive. He said that he masturbated multiple times thinking of her. The murmurs of the sea make him think of the murmurs, the sighs, and the cries of women during sexual relations. The actress' white dress makes him think of the lovely white dresses that his mother used to often wear in summertime. The scene of hemoptysis, during the kiss, reminds him of a cousin who died of tuberculosis about two years after his mother's death. He adds that he and his brother had been instructed not to tell anyone that their cousin had died of that disease, because it might harm the marriage prospects of the deceased's sister. The patient tells me that after that, and for quite some time, he wondered whether his mother, too, hadn't died of tuberculosis and whether they weren't hiding that from him and his brother.

He then added that after his cousin's death, he wondered whether the cause of his mother's death hadn't been twofold, in the event that his suspicion that his mother masturbated was correct: both his father's violence and his mother's masturbation. Hadn't he been told that masturbation could cause imbecility, tuberculosis, or madness? He adds that at that time, he had a phobia of tuberculosis, which lasted for several years.

I must say that this dream struck me immediately as very important. But I didn't think that it was about to lead us so quickly towards the revelation of the primal scene.

As I am in the habit of asking my patients for further associations when this seems useful or necessary to me, I asked G. T. to associate, beyond the hemoptysis, to the bloodstains he saw on the actress' dress and on his sweater after the young woman fainted.

The patient, after thinking for a few seconds, replied: "I remember that when I was really young, I was very unpleasantly surprised and deeply disturbed when I saw a bloody sanitary napkin for the first time in my life."

I asked him whether he could tell me at what age and under what circumstances he had seen this sanitary napkin.

He replied, after thinking about it for a bit, that he must have been three years old, because it happened when his maid was a woman named Helen, and Helen had left when he was less than four years old, and at that time he and his brother were put in the care of another maid, who was a kind of nursemaid. The patient said that Helen would sometimes change her sanitary napkin in front of him, and he added that once he had asked her why she had blood on her genitals. G. T. cannot remember her reply.

"So," I said to him, "you had already seen, at the age of three, the genitals of your maid—meaning one year before you saw the genitals of the little girl who used to play with you, when you were four."

"Indeed," said the patient, and he remained silent for some time. I left him in his silence, and then, after some time, I asked him if he used to sleep in the same room as his maid at that time.

The patient answered that he didn't sleep in the same room as his maid, but rather in the same room as his brother, and that the maid slept in a small adjacent room, and she always left the door open.

I drew Giannis T.'s attention to the idyllic scene at the start of the dream, in which, while he is caressing the American actress' breasts, he is listening to the sighing of the tide, and I ask him whether he hadn't seen and heard something from the adjacent room.

The patient replies immediately: "Certainly yes . . . now I remember a whole scene . . ."

One summer night, he was awakened by a faint noise and sees, in the glow of the nightlight, the door, which usually stayed wide open, softly closing. His brother was asleep. He comes to attention; he hears whispers. Frightened, he gets out of bed and knocks at the door. The maid comes in and closes the door behind her. He tells her that he is afraid and asks her why she closed the door. G. T. does not remember what the maid answered, but he knows that she quietly scolded him and told him to get back to sleep immediately. She put him back into bed and told him that there was no reason to be afraid; she stayed with him for a while and then went back into her own room and locked the door with the key. The patient could not fall back asleep; he was listening. Everything was silent at first. Then he heard whispering again and, sometime after, sighs. Both rooms opened onto a small terrace.

Giannis T. then went out of the door that opened onto the terrace. The maid's words had reassured him. He went towards the door of the maid's room, which also opened onto the terrace, and through the crack between the two shutters of the half-opened door, he saw, in the light of the oil lamp burning on a little table in front of an icon near the bed, a man making love to his maid. The man was standing up, and the maid was lying down flat on the bed, her head on a pillow against the wall. Her nightshirt was lifted up, her thighs were wide open and up in the air, and her knees were bent. And as the man penetrated her, she was sighing and murmuring impassioned words. The man's activity and the state in which he saw the maid terrified the little boy. He watched, stupefied and trembling. Suddenly, the man pulled out and the patient saw his penis, which seemed enormous to him, spurting forth semen onto the maid's belly or thighs.

Following this tale, the patient remained silent for a few moments, and then, after telling me that he now wondered how he, who had such a good memory, could have forgotten this scene, which was obviously of capital importance, he added:

> I now remember that after witnessing this scene, which must have been the prototype of all of my latter sadomasochistic fantasies, I felt seized with terror and standing there, on the terrace, I burst into tears. Helen (the maid) came out to me a short time after and, understanding that I had seen everything, she took me into her room and told me, I believe, that that man was going to be her husband. Then she added that if I promised not to tell anyone, she would be very nice to me, but if I spoke, she or her fiancé would certainly cut off my penis.

With this discovery, we had just made an enormous step forward.

I regret not having had the time to include in this case study my verification of the patient's age at that time, the identity of the maid, and the period of time during which she served G. T.'s family, or to present some of the elements that help explain the patient's "forgetting."

Unfortunately, the length that this paper has taken on does not allow me to enter into these interesting details, nor to present the interpretation I made, the following day, of the last dream, and the patient's associations on that day. The primal scene, which had so long been forgotten, had finally returned to consciousness. The patient, who had initially considered his father's coitus with the chambermaid Maria to have been the "primal scene," from that day on properly named the scene with the maid Helen and her "fiancé" as the "true primal scene."

A relatively short time after this great dénouement in the psychoanalytic treatment of G. T., the patient began to make much more rapid progress. The premature ejaculations became much less premature, and a short time after, G. T. finally managed to ejaculate within the vagina after having made some movements, which though certainly still insufficient in duration, nonetheless it was inside the vagina.

Nonetheless, the premature ejaculations reappeared when Giannis T., who had gradually stopped frequenting prostitutes, and who had finally successfully courted a young woman, made several unsuccessful attempts at deflowering her. In despair, the young man thought that all of the work that had been accomplished to date was crumbling away. But the analytic work continued, and I succeeded in getting Giannis to understand the meaning of this relapse. I should also have liked to present this part of the analysis, which lasted for several months, but, due to the aforementioned time constraints, I am unable do so.

After these last months of analytic work, G. T. succeeded in deflowering the young virgin he had made his mistress. His erections were good, and the duration of the act normal, without ever having exceeded, at least during the analysis, the lower bound of the average duration of normal intercourse. He and his girlfriend nonetheless seemed satisfied.

Giannis T. was also able to work normally and, instead of remaining the subordinate of the lawyer who was employing him as an assistant, became his partner. Towards the end of the treatment, which lasted several more months, the young man, who was now able to compete normally with his brother and his father, told me that although he hadn't stopped being interested in literature or philosophy, he intended to open his own law firm.

Notes

1 Originally published in French as Andreas Embiricos, "Un cas de névrose obsessionnelle avec éjaculations précoces," *Revue Française de Psychanalyse* 14, no. 3 (1950): 331–66.
2 While pretending to be asleep, during school vacations Giannis had twice or thrice observed his brother masturbating in bed. He was around 10 years old at the time; his brother, 14.
3 Karl Abraham, "Ejaculatio Præcox," in *Selected Papers of Karl Abraham, M.D.*, trans. Douglas Bryan and Alix Strachey (London: Hogarth Press, 1927), 280–98, here 286–8.
4 Translator's note: At this point in the original, there is a footnote that specifies: "Greek uses an entirely unrelated word for *entr'acte*." Although the word *entr'acte* is uncommon in English, which uses the word *intermission*, I have kept *entr'acte* from the original not only because Embiricos' subsequent interpretation depends on the presence of the word *act* in both, but also because the use of the word *intermission* in the translation might create an inopportune association in the reader's mind, as it is lacking in the original, with the word *intromission*.

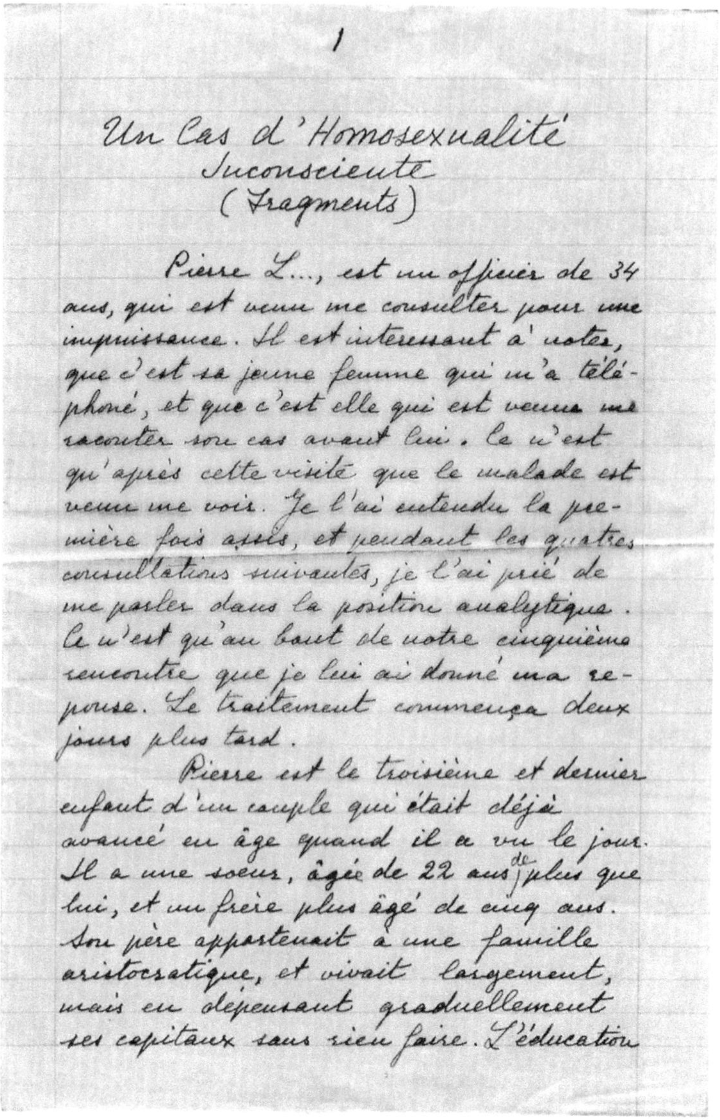

1

Un Cas d'Homosexualité
Inconsciente
(Fragments)

Pierre L..., est un officier de 34 ans, qui est venu me consulter pour une impuissance. Il est interessant à noter, que c'est sa jeune femme qui m'a téléphoné, et que c'est elle qui est venue me raconter son cas avant lui. Ce n'est qu'après cette visite que le malade est venu me voir. Je l'ai entendu la première fois assis, et pendant les quatres consultations suivantes, je l'ai prié de me parler dans la position analytique. Ce n'est qu'au bout de notre cinquième rencontre que je lui ai donné ma réponse. Le traitement commença deux jours plus tard.

Pierre est le troisième et dernier enfant d'un couple qui était déjà avancé en âge quand il a vu le jour. Il a une soeur, âgée de 22 ans de plus que lui, et un frère plus âgé de cinq ans. Son père appartenait à une famille aristocratique, et vivait largement, mais en dépensant graduellement ses capitaux sans rien faire. L'éducation

Figure 2.1 The first page of Andreas Embiricos' French manuscript of the study "A Case of Unconscious Homosexuality" (fair copy written in red ink).

Chapter 2

A Case of Unconscious Homosexuality (Fragments)

Petros L . . ., a thirty-four-year-old military officer, came to consult me for impotence. It is noteworthy that it was his young wife who first telephoned me and came to tell me about the case before he did. Only after this visit did the patient come to see me himself. During our initial meeting, I listened to him while he was seated; during the following four consultations, I asked him to speak to me in the analytic position. It was only at the end of our fifth meeting that I gave him my reply. Treatment began two days later.

Petros is the third and youngest child of a couple who were already advanced in years when he came into the world. He has a sister twenty-two years his senior, and a brother, also older than he, though only by five years. His father came from an aristocratic family and lived lavishly, though gradually spending down his capital without ever doing any work. Petros' education was markedly deficient and inadequate. In later years, he sought—with considerable success—to remedy these shortcomings through independent study, which he pursued in addition to his military training, before entering the army as a career officer. He was quite literally brought up "in the folds of his mother's skirts" and became passionately attached to her. His mother, who never allowed him to eat meat, instilled in him lofty ideals of a vaguely Deistic nature and tried to inculcate beliefs akin to those of Christian Science. Petros had very little contact with his father and, besides playing some sports, he led a largely idle life. His mother, unwilling to send him to school at the usual age, insisted he keep his hair long and treated him more or less as though he were a little girl. It should also be noted that Petros slept in his mother's bed until the age of ten and that throughout that entire period he had no bed of his own. When he was six, a governess once threw pepper into his eyes. Around the same time, while his mother was reading him a story, he experienced the uncanny sensation of seeing two gnomes appear before him.

Up until the age of eight, Petros loved his mother more than anyone else. But he was also passionately attached to a little niece of his own age, Helen, who lived with them until the age of ten. The two children were inseparable. They used to play together and, among their other games, they enjoyed killing mosquitos, collecting dried animal droppings from the garden and the woods, and hiding together behind sofas, armchairs, or beneath tables, imagining that they were building little houses or nests in each of these places.

During his childhood, Petros liked to torment animals, and once even tried to crush some kittens. I should also add that, from time to time, he amused himself by pulling the braids of his father's chauffeur's little girl, at a time when he himself still wore his hair long, like a young girl.

He was ashamed of this long hair, which he did not cut short until the age of ten or twelve. At times, he would wear a handkerchief on his head to conceal his long hair as best he could. But his mother insisted that he keep it long all those years. She also wished to make him a vegetarian. For his part, he too long wished to keep his long hair, despite the shame he felt, and was terrified at the thought that it might one day be cut off.

I shall underscore one further important factor before moving on to memories belonging to a later period in my patient's life. Throughout the whole of Petros' childhood and adolescence, his father appears to have played an elusive role, one far removed from that of a normal father. It was a family friend, an army general and loyal companion of his mother, who seems to have fulfilled the function of a true father figure, although it was always the mother who held the predominant place in family life. The general was markedly more masculine in temperament and demeanor than the patient's father and it was he who contributed more than anyone else to the eventual decision to have the boy's long hair cut.

The period of Petros' great love for his mother lasted until his eighth year. Around that time, his mother began to turn increasingly toward Pavlos, the elder brother, and to show a growing interest in this son, who was then thirteen. She would often shut herself away with him, and they would converse together at length. She took a keen interest in everything Pavlos did (amongst other things, music) and began to neglect her younger son. Petros suffered deeply from this change and recalls this period with great sorrow, as it marked the waning of his passionate attachment to his mother.

My patient felt himself inferior to his brother, with whom he had nothing in common. At the same time, he nourished the hope of becoming strong like him, of surpassing him, or at least of becoming his equal; yet this desire filled him with great apprehension and aroused a profound anxiety.

He began to masturbate at the age of twelve or thirteen, he continues to do so to this day. He also resorts to mutual masturbation with his wife, with whom he does not even dare to attempt coitus. He is extraordinarily dependent upon this young woman and cannot bear, even for a moment, to be deprived of what she represents for him. Only after several weeks of analysis did he begin to understand more clearly that he desires his wife as a mother who dispenses all satisfactions. He wishes to derive pleasure from her passively and seeks in her not a lover or a wife, but an active creator of voluptuous pleasures, an inexhaustible nurturing mother, a powerful protectress. The slightest delay on her part in understanding his profoundly troubled emotional states, the slightest disappointment in the fulfillment of his expectations, plunges him into a more or less intense anxiety. Despite his gentle nature, he is extremely impatient with her; despite his desire to make her happy, he is capriciously demanding. Although he does love her, it is easy to see that he loves her only in relation to his profound narcissism. Before undergoing analytic treatment, Petros could not imagine that his wife's languor and occasional sadness might stem from a lack of genuine fulfillment.

Before his marriage, while masturbating, Petros would sometimes envision slaughterhouse scenes and animals being killed; more often, however, his masturbatory fantasies involved pretty girls or beautiful women. At times, he would engage in masturbation while looking at photographs or illustrations of young girls, imagining that he was exchanging kisses and caresses with them, though never imagining performing coitus with them. He also derived great satisfaction from looking at old fashion magazines, and even more so from seeing, touching, trying on, and wearing his mother's corsets and other feminine garments.

His first sexual experience, or rather his first contact, with a young woman took place at the age of eighteen. The young woman was a maidservant in his father's household, and he spent several nights with her in her bed. He experienced erections, but did everything he could to conceal them, because he was felt ashamed and believed it was sinful to reveal his penis, whether erect or not, and that it was even more sinful to use one's penis to obtain pleasure from a woman. It was only barely, and with great difficulty, that he dared to touch the young servant girl's breasts during the nights he spent with her. Naturally, he felt the same sense of guilt regarding masturbation, although with the difference that, when he was alone, he was nevertheless able to carry out the masturbatory act to completion.

Yet we must return to the patient's childhood memories in order to fully understand his emotional development and his complexual organization. Despite a few dark clouds, Petros appears to have been relatively happy up until the age of eight. It was at that time that two events occurred, two events he regards as the beginning of his later difficulties.

First: his mother began at that time to favor his brother Pavlos. Second: little Helen, who had previously shown him warm affection, began around the same period to act coldly towards him.

All of his efforts to win back little Helen's love proved in vain. Disheartened, he stopped showing her any affection and, in the end, not only did he cease to love her, but quarreled with her as well.

To console himself, he turned to his toys. During that rather extended period, he tried to imitate his brother Pavlos, whom he continued to regard, with a painful sense of inferiority, as a very strong and greatly superior boy.

At the age of fifteen, Petros began to display mystical aspirations of a somewhat pantheistic kind and experienced powerful surges of love for nature. At the same time, despite his mounting feelings of guilt and anxiety, he engaged in masturbation with increasing frequency. One may infer that, as his anxiety became eroticized, it in turn became a source of masochistic gratification. By the age of eighteen, the mystical tendencies had waned, but the masturbation persisted.

It should be noted that, despite his timidity, anxiety, and hypersensitivity, and despite his feeling of inferiority (or, rather, because of that feeling), Petros aspired to become, and in fact did become, a military officer like his mother's friend, the general. In this way, he sought to use that counterweight to compensate for and offset as far as possible, the deficiencies created in him by his sense of inferiority. He began his studies at home and later attended a preparatory school; during this period, he also took up athletics in order to develop his body and become strong.

He eventually resolved to change his way of life and began seeking out the company of women, attempting to become something of a libertine and affecting a certain amorality. Yet, beneath all these masks he remained inwardly withdrawn, timid, and above all, deeply anxious, never daring to make love with a woman, and still less to deflower a virgin.

Despite his difficulties, Petros succeeded in his military studies and became an officer shortly before the war, in which he later served not on the battlefield but in the military administration, where he was promoted to the rank of major.

In the army, where he has remained, he is regarded as a capable officer; yet he suffers deeply from his impotence and anxiety, and feels himself inept and inadequate in the performance of his duties as a soldier. He finds it very difficult to command others, though he manages, through exhausting effort, to conceal his inner state and to maintain appearances with both his subordinates and his superiors.

Between 1941 and 1942, he came to believe that his only remaining course was to flee the world, change his way of life, and become a priest in order to escape the anxiety provoked in him by rivalry with men and the demands of life. He did not enter the priesthood, but he did convert to Catholicism, which had fascinated him during the preceding years. Yet the idea of becoming a priest continued to haunt him and did not leave him until he resolved to marry, hoping that married life might help him overcome his impotence. This hope proved vain, and shortly after his marriage he consulted two or three physicians in search of a remedy, but the treatments they prescribed were of no avail. His impotence persisted, and his entire attitude toward his young wife (as, indeed, toward the other women he had known before her) remained that of a young girl who loves another girl homosexually.

Finally, a colleague advised him to undergo analysis and recommended that he come to see me, which Petros did about a year after his marriage, telling me, amongst other things, that he feared he was "devoid of sexual instincts." After seeing him several times, I tried to explain his case to him in psychoanalytic terms, and he decided to undertake analytic treatment.

* * *

One must suspect, beneath Petros L . . .'s symptoms of anxiety and other reactions, a totally unconscious homosexuality. The patient is profoundly fixated upon his mother, and his libido seeks satisfactions in a pregenital manner, along oral and anal lines. The Oedipal complex is inverted. From an etiological standpoint, the psychological situation is determined by the patient's identification with his mother, the introjection of the fraternal threat, and an intense castration anxiety. This state of affairs conditions the complete reversal of Petros' Oedipal complex: in assuming the role of a castrated being in everyday life, he desires to obtain what his mother receives from his father, namely the penis, so as to be able to enjoy it passively, as a woman would. The entire complexual *status quo* of the patient lends his neurosis a clearly narcissistic character.

The Dream

The following dream, with its interpretation, illustrates Petros' case and sheds light on both the content and the structure of his neurosis. The patient had this dream close to the start of the third month of his treatment.

> I was dressed elegantly. I was wearing my finest suit, of which I was proud, and I was waiting to go out to some evening party in the company of certain people, one of whom seemed to be Helen (the patient's niece) and another Pavlos (his elder brother). Although I had the impression that Pavlos was there, I was not certain of his presence. I was smoking a cigarette and the ash kept falling onto my suit, burning it, which worried me, though I did not stop smoking. Suddenly, I dropped my cigarette onto my suit and began to search for it, but without success. I did not feel overly ashamed, although I knew that what I was doing was out of the ordinary. At first, I felt rather confident and self-possessed, but then I became increasingly anxious and miserable when I realized that I had just made a large black burn near the upper part of my trousers, and that this burn spread across the buttons. The buttons had also turned black. I wanted then more than ever to look my best, so I took my ivory brush and began frantically brushing the burnt area. Some black powder flew into the air, leaving stains on the brush. The more I brushed the burnt spot, the blacker the powder became, and I realized that there was no longer any hope. It was at that moment that I saw my wife and her sister, who was about the same age as she. Both were dressed very elegantly, also for an evening gathering. They were walking down a path toward their mother, who was waiting to choose the more beautiful of the two. I realized that both were absolutely beautiful. My wife was wearing a cluster of grapes at her waist. The grapes were a creamy color, and suddenly I noticed that the grapes at the lower part of each cluster were crushed and that all the grapes were covered in

dust. I knew that this was a terrible tragedy that would greatly pain my wife. Because of this, she could not appear as beautiful as she otherwise would have.

My wife approached the body of water nearby and she lay down in such a way that her hair and the grapes were immersed in the water, with which she was trying to wash away the dust, and also attempting to restore the crushed grapes. At the same time, she said in an anguished voice that seemed to echo within my head and that I still heard upon awakening: "We must make love! We must make love!"

The Patient's Associations

1. "The water reminds me of the pond near our country property, which, as a child, I once saw a little girl fall into. I felt a certain sexual-type attraction toward that little girl, yet at the same time I felt critical of her. The little girl was unharmed as a result of her fall."
2. "The burns remind me of my brother Pavlos."
3. "The grapes remind me of young Helen. This association carries for me a feeling of desolation."

The Analyst's Interpretation

Petros is dressed elegantly like the ladies, and he is in competition with them. Pavlos, his brother, is a stand-in for the father. The patient says has the impression that he sees his brother, but is not certain of his presence. I explained to him that when he says that Pavlos is there, he places him before himself, not in order to compete with him, but to charm him, and that when he says he is uncertain of his presence, it is because he wants to distance him in order to evade a dangerous enemy whom he wants to eliminate, but whom he is afraid of confronting, so that he may remain alone in passive enjoyment of their mother. This shows that he does not want to accept the consequences (namely, rivalry) arising from an identification of his genitals with those of his father and of his father's substitute, Pavlos, since for him, any rivalry with the father would entail castration.

The cigarette that Petros smokes symbolizes both the maternal breast and the penis. I explained to him that he treats the breast as a penis not only because he wishes to obtain gratification from both, but also because he seeks to compensate for the anxiety-inducing absence of a virile organ in his mother (whom he regards as having been castrated by his father) by imaginatively endowing her with one. In this way, he also expresses, alongside his desire to enjoy both the penis and the breast, the wish to restore his mother (and, through his identification with her, to restore himself) by conceiving of the breasts as possessing, in addition to their natural meaning as feminine attributes, a phallic or masculine significance.

In this attitude, one can discern the mechanism of the feeling of omnipotence and the nostalgia for that omnipotence, not only through the denial of reality, but also through the desire to incorporate, orally and anally, both the breast and the penis.

By smoking the cigarette, that is by sucking at the breast-penis, Petros let fall (or flow) onto his clothing the ash-milk-semen. This troubles the patient. He feels anxious because he experiences guilt over having derived pleasure from both the breast and the penis, and because he wished not only to make use of these organs but also to tear them away from their possessors and make them his own through incorporation. He is also anxious because he feels guilty about his masturbation, fearing that by carrying out the masturbatory act he may lose his penis (and with it his semen and his health) and be castrated.

His trousers are burnt in several places. He castrates himself as punishment and so as not to lose the love of his mother and father. In exchange for this sacrifice of his virility, he demands the penis and the breast so that he may enjoy them passively and fill the void left by the burns. Yet despite his anxiety, he continues to smoke and to burn his clothing. I explained to Petros that, having inflicted this punishment upon himself, he thereby grants himself the right to continue deriving passive pleasure, and I added that his worry (anxiety) has become eroticized and that he draws from it a masochistic pleasure which he prolongs by continuing to burn his clothing while smoking, thus turning his sadism not against the father or the brother, but against himself. In this way he becomes a victim—that is to say, according to the sadistic conception of the sexual act, a woman—a victim-woman at the disposal of the phallic men and women whom he desires and whose love he seeks.

I explained to Petros that when, in the dream, he lets his cigarette fall and searches for it without finding it, the reason it remains unfindable is that he has ingested (incorporated) it—made it disappear like a penis that he has taken into himself. The cigarette is contained within the burn-hole. In this way, he tears it away from his father through the paternal substitute of his brother Pavlos (who, lest we forget, is both present and absent in the dream). He absorbs the cigarette, thereby enacting simultaneously the incorporation into the burn-hole and the anal castration of his brother-father.

Petros also says, in recounting his dream, that he does not feel too ashamed when he notices the ladies thinking about him. He does not feel overly ashamed because he is, in effect, competing with them, having absorbed the cigarette-penis just as women ingest men's sexual organ. In this way, he turns his back on the reality that provokes his anxiety, and he feels powerful through the presence of the penis within him, a situation from which he draws compensation for his impotence. It is as though he were saying to the women: "See, I do the same as you—and even better than you, for I keep the penis inside of myself permanently (in my burn-hole, my anus), whereas you are less skilled as I am at taking men's penises from them with your vaginas, your anuses, and your mouths." This explains why he feels confident and independent after the disappearance of the cigarette: confident = strong through captation, having retained the penis inside of him, just as he retains his feces; independent, in that he has no need of heterosexual relations nor of competing with other men for the conquest of women.

But soon afterward, he feels anxious and very unhappy upon realizing that the ash has left a large burn extending over the buttons and the upper part of his trousers. I interpret this reaction as follows:

The burn is too big for the penis to have been left behind; the buttons are gone, the trousers are left open, and Petros runs the risk of letting the incorporated penis escape. But, without it, he feels exposed to the danger of having to assert his own organ, which is, in his eyes, cut off, castrated, or so small in comparison to his father's or his brother's that it has no meaning other than that of a sort of insignificant vestige of a once-normal penis that has been removed. He considers it, in his anxiety, to be analogous to what he would see in contemplating a woman's genitalia: the clitoris uselessly perched above the much larger orifice of the vulva, both of which represent for him the voluptuous yet horrifying remnants of the castrating intervention of the powerful, sadistic father.

But Petros tells us that in his dream he wanted more than ever to look his best. That is why he takes an ivory brush and frenetically brushes the gaping burn. I explained to him that, in brushing himself, he is furiously masturbating. He uses the brush to pleasure himself with anxiety-voluptuousness-orgasm, since, for him, the female orgasm, like his own, amounts to anxiety, meaning it is a sadomasochistic pleasure. He wishes to attain that state, and through it to reach the apogee of pleasure, which for him coincides with what he feels at the height of his anxiety, seeking to attain climax by this means, just as he imagines that women (those who are not phallic) do.

At the same time, this very gesture allows him to appease the demands of his superego (the introjected paternal threats), for by brushing himself he seeks to remove the traces of his id's drive activity and to restore balance through expiation. He regards his anal and oral eroticism—particularly their sadistic and aggressive manifestations—as well as his masturbatory pleasures, as profoundly shameful. He also acts in this way in order to earn the right, after punishment, to begin anew the full cycle of pleasure-seeking in the passive-homosexual mode, being unable to accept his positive Oedipus complex.

A bit of powder from the charred fabric of his trousers flies off and stains the brush, but the burn remains large and black, and he cannot make it disappear. When he says in his dream, "there was no longer any hope . . ." he means that there was no hope of incorporating the penis in a definitive and permanent way, as in an eternal mystical union.

In other words, we may conclude that, in the frenetic masturbation of this dream, as in all of his waking masturbations, Petros L . . . seeks not only to passively take pleasure from his mother, but also, by feeling and experiencing all of her sensations, to take pleasure from his father's penis as she does.

Indeed, he imaginarily receives within himself, through his identification with his mother, all of the repercussions of the father's coitus, of which he thus becomes the passionate recipient and the ardent libidinal object, thereby realizing the roles of both parents while taking himself as his own object.

Further on in this dream, Petros' rivalry with his mother and her substitutes becomes more apparent, as do his reactions towards his analyst.

> It was at that moment that I saw my wife and her sister, who was about the same age as she. Both of were dressed very elegantly, also for an evening gathering. They were walking down a path toward their mother, who was waiting to choose the more beautiful of the two. I realized that both were absolutely beautiful. My wife was wearing a cluster of grapes at her waist. The grapes were a creamy color, and suddenly I noticed that the grapes at the lower part of each cluster were crushed . . .

I interpreted this passage of the dream as follows.

Being much too afraid of confronting his father and Pavlos, of rivaling them for his mother and his wife, and unable to live, as he would have wished, in the continual realization within himself of both the maternal and paternal roles, Petros unconsciously resolves to be nothing more than a woman in his passivity. From that moment on, he ceases to act in the dream and becomes an absolutely passive spectator, while his wife takes the initiative.

The grapes that she wears in her hair and at her waist symbolize the penis that Petros wishes his wife had in reality and with which he equips her in the dream, thereby expressing his desire that she might become a phallic woman and his wish to find in her a male lover. Yet, unfortunately for him, his wife does not value the penis-grapes he gives her. This signifies the resentment Petros feels, both in waking life and in the dream, that his wife remains a woman rather than possessing a penis and acting like a man. The crushed grapes at the lower portions of the clusters indicate that she is castrated. She has only a clitoris (the remnant of a severed penis) and a vagina, she remains a woman nonetheless, whereas the patient's mother seems to have been, in both behavior and her character, a phallic woman. In his dream, as in reality, Petros is deeply dissatisfied that his young wife does not perform the masculine role he expected of her.

The bunches of grapes are cream-colored, a hue evocative of both milk and semen, whose emission may be brought about through sucking, coitus, or masturbation (a nostalgic allusion to the sucking of the breasts, the oral sucking of the penis, the drawing-in of the penis by the vagina, masturbatory friction, and the pressure and contractions of the anal sphincter). The fact that the grapes are crushed in the dream also signifies that Petros is distressed that his wife, in reality as in the dream, does not emit milk or semen from her clitoris or urethra, and that his wife, as a castrated being, is unable to offer him the satisfactions he desires from her.

Petros also says in his dream that he knows that everything taking place constitutes a great tragedy. Indeed, the fact that his wife sought in him a husband, a lover, a man—and not a sister—when she took him to be her husband is a great tragedy. But, it is his own tragedy that Petros expresses through his wife's tragedy, since, by identifying with her, he awaits from her a virile love he has never been able to find in reality, as his homosexuality has always been unconscious and conflicted. Because of this tragedy, his wife cannot appear as beautiful as she otherwise would have, as he himself remarks in the dream.

But all of that is nothing but a phase in Petros' progression toward complete identification with his wife. In the next scene, total identification takes place. It is Petros who, in fact, *is* this beautiful woman with the crushed grapes and the castrated penis. It is he who lies down by the water (his mother's water) and, when he says that his wife (that is to say, himself) strives in vain to wash and restore the smashed grapes, he is expressing through this scene his fear of leaving his mother's breast, of becoming a man, of being cured by regaining his phallus and virile potency. He is also expressing, through his wish to crawl back inside his mother's body, the wish to experience, in complete receptivity and passivity, the sexual (coital) activity of the father by means of the mother. It is he who will experience her pleasures, by incorporating himself into her, by reintegrating himself into her, by becoming one with her body, by becoming himself the mother whom the father can possess.

The dream ends with a frenzied appeal that Petros is addressing to his analyst through his wife's mouth. He utters this appeal like a cry of burning desire, and at the same time, a cry of distress and anxiety (that is to say, for Petros, a profoundly voluptuous cry), which, as he reports, continued to resonate in his head even after awakening: "We must make love! We must make love!"

I translate the language of his unconscious as follows: "My analyst, my analytic father, do not speak to me of restoring my penis or competing with you for the conquest of women . . . Give me your penis instead . . . Come and penetrate me through the mouth and through the anus . . . Otherwise, I shall spend my whole life masturbating if you ask me to become a man and to copulate with women . . ."

Chapter 3

Psychoanalytic Technique[1]

Ladies and Gentlemen

In our previous sessions, I described to you how psychoanalysis was born; I laid out for you the main axes of its theory, which was gradually created and constituted by the genius of Freud over the course of the long and fertile years of his gigantic labor. Today, I shall speak to you about psychoanalytic technique, without which this initiation—intended for those who wish to learn about psychoanalysis otherwise than from summary vulgarizations or irresponsible ramblings—would not be complete. This way, you will be able to form your own ideas about what psychoanalysis is. Perhaps in the future some of you will want to undertake further study in order to participate (and there are many ways of doing so) in this grand movement that bears within it absolutely certain possibilities of a future total renewal of this world. Because, as I explained in my first talk, although psychoanalysis began as a new form of therapy, it quickly became a theory of cosmic dimensions, whose goals incommensurably surpass the boundaries of psychotherapy and the prophylaxis of the neuroses, a worldview whose goals lie far beyond the limits of humanity's current possibilities. These goals shall constitute the subject of my next and last talk, which will conclude this brief series of introductory discussions.

Psychoanalytic technique was not always what it is today. Throughout time, technique has reflected the different stages of psychoanalysis' development and the discoveries that had been made at each period of our young science's theoretical and practical evolution. As I cannot describe to you all of the phases through which this technique passed before becoming the perfected instrument that it currently is, without sacrificing the space required for a concise and summary presentation of its current form, I shall leave aside the initial approaches and various phases of its evolution (which you are able to surmise to a certain extent from what I previously told you in a much more detailed fashion about the evolution of theory) in order to describe to you what analysts do today (and when I use the term *analyst*, I always mean the orthodox Freudian analyst) in order to treat their patients, taking as my basis firstly the teaching of Freud, and then the work of some of his disciples, such as Sándor Ferenczi, René Laforgue, and Edward Glover.

As you have already heard, analysis has nothing in common with suggestion, exhortation, moralization, psychotherapeutics, or with those recent "panaceas" known as narcoanalysis and electroshock.

Psychoanalysis is a therapeutic based on a concrete theory of the drives and their conflicts, on the existence of the unconscious, on the global and dynamic concept of the individual and universal libido, and on the psychobiological concept of the organization of the human psyche. These were brought to light by the discovery of the powers that are deeply at work within the unconscious—the unconscious which was so well explored, understood, and described by Sigmund Freud.

This is therefore quite far removed from what ordinary psychotherapists do: they base their work on static and arbitrary principles and on data that they hold are derived from the conscious layer of human personality, or, at the very most, its pre-conscious layer; however, the true determinants of the various phenomena that patients present originate in the unconscious, which is something that totally eludes these traditional psychotherapists.

In psychoanalysis, we adopt a wholly different approach. We seek to reach the unconscious in order to explore it and to find within it the true keys to complexes. We can use these keys in order to gradually resolve the conflicts and problems that gave birth to our patients' neuroses or personality disorders. We cause them to relive their conflicts with us in a way that eventually becomes conscious, within the analytic situation which I summarized for you in our earlier discussions, by using what I have already described to you; namely, transference. It is through the transference that we make our patients' unconscious material conscious. We accomplish this work through the emotional repercussions of our interpretative elaborations—not by a sort of catechism addressed to our patients' intellect. You will recall the phenomenon I named resistance. Well, it is impossible to overcome a complex without overcoming the specific phenomena that constantly reappear in a treatment, without making them conscious, too, which will eventually allow our patients to realize themselves by finding their own way of reconciling and harmonizing, within themselves and as members of society, the pleasure principle with the reality principle.

But the difference that separates us radically from ordinary psychotherapists does not only reside within what I have just said. By means of this long collaboration—hindered from its outset by the resistances, and transformed, in a way, into a sort of collaborative struggle rather than a collaboration, properly speaking, but which is the only one that will allow for the defeat of the neurosis—we reconstitute, on new bases, not our patients' personalities, which we cannot change and which we do not seek to change, but rather the economy of their psychic organization. In other words, we help them gradually to be able to synthesize, on their own, the forces that make up their psychic personality, which is the same as providing new foundations for the intrapsychic relationships and interplay between their Ego, their Id, and their Super-Ego, by making the action of the latter as flexible, as harmless, and as un-reactionary as possible, and by removing its unconscious character as much as possible, without which we will not be able to perform the cure, or, at least, to achieve a considerable and lasting improvement.

Let us imagine that the patient is a State undergoing a profound crisis. The ordinary psychotherapist will attempt to overcome this crisis by replacing the government, but he or she will leave the deficient status quo that existed within the State absolutely intact, meaning that he or she will do nothing to discover, understand, and liquidate the true causes of the crisis. These therapists not only cannot remedy—they do not even see the causes of the problem. And should a few of them speculate, to a certain extent, where this crisis originates, they have neither the courage nor the means to deal with the situation, mainly because they bear these same conflicts in their own unconscious, in perhaps an attenuated and better-repressed form, but sufficiently intact to make them incapable of dealing with their patients' problems. This is why, because they fear their own conflicts (by this, we mean the fear of seeing clearly within themselves their own sexual problems and their own instincts, which form the basis of all successive, rationalized crises), they react towards their patients as they would react towards their own unconscious tendencies, and they attempt to perform cures by dictating decrees *ex cathedra*, which are nothing more than formulas devoid of meaning, and which are often quite harmful or even sometimes comically puerile.

They do not see that even a good government cannot resolve a profound crisis without changing the ailing constitution of that State, and without affecting the broken articulation of its institutions and its outdated laws; in sum, without globally changing the previous status quo—evidently in such cases where this status quo is the true reason for the societal or national problem.

So, these therapists fail in their efforts, exceptional individuals though they may be.

Psychoanalysis adopts an entirely different approach. It does not change the government of this ailing State. It does not cling to the naïve idea that repression, force, idealization, or fatalism are capable of offering solutions. It does not wish to appoint a dictator. Rather, it entrusts the task of replacing the government, when this is necessary, with the forces that become liberated (be they revolutionary forces) and which will emerge from the therapeutic process of analysis to form the new, natural government at the right time.[2]

The psychoanalyst is not this government. He is an important and necessary power, dispassionate yet profoundly present and, as the personification of this power, he observes the conflict neither as an arbiter, nor as a spectator, but as a trainer of the liberated revolutionary forces that he uses in a certain way (let us emphasize that he remains passive) and for a special purpose: his goal is that the outcome of the struggle shall be the reintegration of these living forces (the freed and eventually genital libido) into the State, but in a way that allows the State to continue to exist biologically as part of the international community, able to accept rivalry with others, creating its own independent *modus vivendi*, with its own way of attaining its desires without falling back into crisis, without flight into utopia, but truly and in reality, by the gradual positivization and valorization of its creative forces, meaning by Eros and when necessary by conflict with others.

Far from being a dictator, the psychoanalyst becomes, in a sense, at the same time: a trainer, a sort of projection, and a prolongation of the battlefield, and always takes care not to substitute the patient's personality with his own.

A task such as this cannot be accomplished by persons who are not sufficiently protected against the danger of becoming champions, personally fulfilling the desires of the patient (positive countertransference) or enemies of their affectivity (negative countertransference). The psychoanalyst, in order to accomplish his difficult and often thankless task, must remain a disciplined and aware *agent provocateur*, and (in my opinion, which is also that of the majority of Freudian analysts) he must remain, except in rare cases and in rare circumstances, absolutely passive to the end, limiting himself to helping his patients to liquidate their conflicts and to become capable of realizing themselves on their own in actuality. In other words, the primary condition which is necessary in order to be able to perform true analyses is for the analyst to have been thoroughly analyzed himself.

That said, let us now move on to the question of analytic technique.

After the consultation, which often extends beyond the first appointment or two, and once a diagnosis has been made, the treatment begins, excepting in certain cases about which we have doubts: we only take such cases on a trial basis, in order to determine whether or not the analytic method may be applied to them.

In the first session, we set down the conditions and ask the analysand to comply with the fundamental rule: to say everything that comes into his mind literally, to bring us all of his dreams, daydreams, and fantasies, to accept our silence when we do not speak to him or when we do not answer him. We tell him how much our fee is for each hour, we set the times of the sessions, which must take place daily except Sundays, and we inform him of how long our vacation is.

The times set aside for the sessions belong to the patient. We explain to him that no absence shall release him from the obligation of paying for his sessions, even if his absence is long, and even if it is due to an illness, for example.

Let us see now how psychoanalytic technique—which I believed is of use to precede by these few pages, and whose contents will make it easier for those of you who have not yet studied analysis—is applied in practice.

The analytic treatment (always via transference) is performed on two levels—either simultaneously or successively, or even in parallel, if you wish. The first is that of the libido; the second, that of the Ego (energy–structure).[3]

Notes

1 This little series of talks is dedicated to René Laforgue, to whom I owe a great part of my analytic, practical, and theoretical knowledge, as well as many other things besides.

2 Princess Marie Bonaparte finds the word "natural" unsuited and proposes rational (utilitarian—impartial).

3 Editor's note: The manuscript ends abruptly at this point.

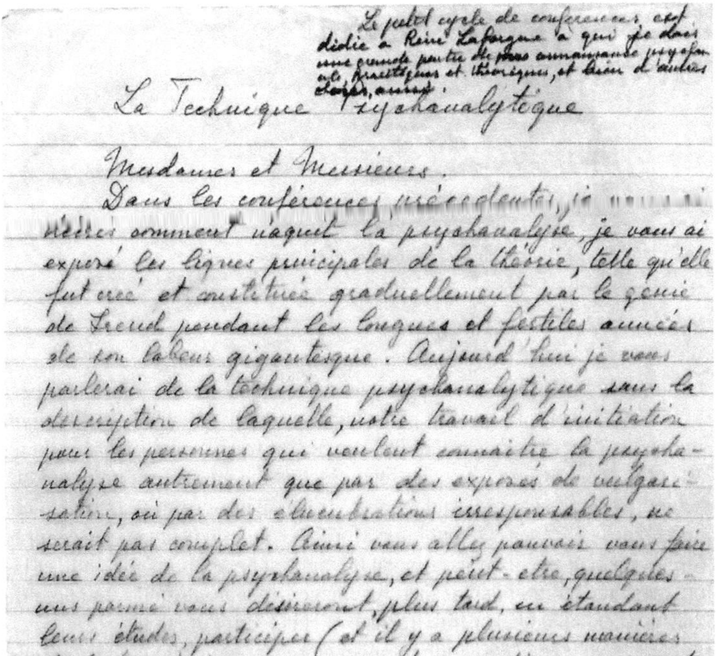
Le petit cycle de conférences est dédié à René Laforgue à qui je dois une grande partie de mes connaissances psychanalytiques pratiques et théoriques, et bien d'autres choses aussi.

La Technique Psychanalytique

Mesdames et Messieurs,

Dans les conférences précédentes, je vous ai décrit comment naquit la psychanalyse, je vous ai exposé les lignes principales de la théorie, telle qu'elle fut créé et constituée graduellement par le génie de Freud pendant les longues et fertiles années de son labeur gigantesque. Aujourd'hui je vous parlerai de la technique psychanalytique sans la description de laquelle, notre travail d'initiation pour les personnes qui veulent connaître la psychanalyse autrement que par des exposés de vulgarisation, ou par des élucubrations irresponsables, ne serait pas complet. Ainsi vous allez pouvoir vous faire une idée de la psychanalyse, et peut-être, quelques-uns parmi vous désireront, plus tard, en étendant leurs études, participer (et il y a plusieurs manières de le faire) à ce mouvement grandiose qui porte en lui des possibilités absolument certaines, d'un renouveau futur total de ce monde. Parce que comme je vous le disais, à ma première conférence, si la psychanalyse a débuté comme une nouvelle thérapeutique, elle est vite devenue une cosmothéorie qui dépasse incommensurablement les cadres de la psychothérapie et de la prophylaxie des névroses, une cosmothéorie dont les buts se trouvent bien au delà des bornes des possibilités actuelles de l'humanité. Ces buts constitueront le sujet de ma prochaine et dernière conférence par laquelle je terminerai ce petit cycle de causeries initiatiques.

La technique psychanalytique ne fut pas toujours ce qu'elle est aujourd'hui. Elle correspondait

Figure 3.1 The first page of Andreas Embiricos' French manuscript of the lecture "Psychoanalytic Technique" (written in pencil, with numerous additions and erasures).

Chapter 4

In Memory of Marie Bonaparte

When, in a familiar wood through which we so often wandered, a great tree is suddenly absent—a tree rich in strong branches, with a dense and beautiful canopy beneath and around which we once breathed its life-giving fragrance—one feels not as though a single tree has been felled, but as though an entire stand of forest has vanished. Such is the magnitude of the void left behind by so great a tree. And then, overcome with sorrow, we strive to conjure it back—or even without effort, for a fleeting moment, we see again before us that tall tree, once rustling at the lightest breath of wind. Until, at last, the harsh recognition dawns that this image is but an illusion—an apparition that, as such, could never truly replace or stand in for the living presence.

Such a void was left within our own close circle of friends and colleagues by the death of Marie Bonaparte, who was also, of course, a Princess of Greece, the wife of Prince George, son of the King.

As a princess of our country, Marie Bonaparte was naturally known to all, beloved and respected. Yet, beyond the borders of our land, throughout the West—in Europe, the Americas, and especially in France—our profoundly democratic princess was even more widely known: as a luminous intellect, a generous heart, a brilliant mind of rare clarity, and a tranquil spirit whose radiant warmth and universal influence elevated her to heights even greater than those conferred by her noble birth and royal titles.

Marie Bonaparte! Who among us does not feel a shiver of emotion and admiration each time your name is spoken? Who among us is not deeply stirred when recalling your image, so strikingly reminiscent of your illustrious ancestor, the First Consul Bonaparte? Who among us does not feel a personal gratitude when remembering how you were always and everywhere present, extending a hand of precious, effective, and freely-given assistance whenever the need arose, to any true friend or collaborator, and not infrequently, even to those who were not truly your friends? How could it be otherwise? How could we not remember you with both emotion and admiration, when you were the one who, alongside Anna Freud and a few other women, stood deservedly amongst the foremost disciples of the new science that revealed the hidden mysteries of the psyche? You stood their equal, at the right hand of Sigmund

Freud, and you too were recognized as a worthy student of the great Master, whose spirit continues to illuminate the world with an unfading light, far beyond the visible horizons of the earth.

In a few weeks, it will be a year since that harsh hour when death took you from us. Now, the light Attic earth covers your ashes, beneath ever-gentle trees, within whose rustling the clear flutes of eternal Pan shall forever echo.

Marie Bonaparte! As the humblest tribute of honor, but also of love, allow that two more titles be added to your memory, two titles indelible. To me, you are Athena Pallas, and at the same time the gentle Lady of Mercy: Athena Pallas, because you fought with wisdom, with spear and shield, not only upon the ramparts of psychoanalytic orthodoxy, but also on the front lines of many other noble struggles; and you are, at once, the Lady of Mercy, of Compassion, for wherever pain howled, or stood silent, pleading only with the eyes, it was your wondrous hand that reached out, Marie, soldier and saint.

Chapter 5

Biographical Note on Marie Bonaparte[1]

Marie Bonaparte was born in France in 1882. She was the daughter of Roland Bonaparte. Her education was broad and wide-ranging, and her intellectual horizon was extraordinarily expansive. She engaged deeply with literature, philosophy, psychology, history, medicine, biology, and—above all—with psychoanalysis, to which she dedicated the most productive years of her life, writing many important psychoanalytic studies and masterfully translating many of Sigmund Freud's writings into French. She was on friendly terms with many distinguished authors, eminent scholars, and political leaders from across the ideological spectrum, and she was thus capable of conversing on all subjects with remarkable knowledge, precision, and objectivity. Amongst her friends were Gustave Le Bon, Aristide Bruant, Jean Rostand, Julius Wagner-Jauregg, and many others with whom she maintained regular correspondence, always writing by hand and with incredible alacrity, never leaving a single letter unanswered, even when it came from a stranger. The most significant of her friendships, nonetheless, was the longstanding and extremely fruitful amity she maintained with Sigmund Freud, the founder of psychoanalysis, of whom she was a distinguished pupil.

Here, it should be noted that when the Nazi persecutions of psychoanalysts began, and Freud himself—both as the father of psychoanalysis and as a Jew—found himself in grave danger, Marie Bonaparte hurried at once to Vienna, where, at her own risk, she stood up to Hitler, Goebbels, and other bloodthirsty National-Socialists with astonishing courage and resolve, and she literally saved the Great Teacher from the clutches of those terrifying beasts, spending substantial sums from her personal fortune to ensure he was able to escape Austria and comfortably resettle in London.

Another testament to Marie Bonaparte's courage, generosity, and inner fortitude was her stance and active participation in the struggles of the first orthodox Greek psychoanalysts during the heroic early years of their activity. When the nascent Greek psychoanalytic group was fighting to establish and disseminate psychoanalysis (by which I mean Orthodox Freudian psychoanalysis) in

Greece, despite immense hardships, misunderstandings, misrepresentations, slander, and hostility, Marie Bonaparte stood in full solidarity with that small but spirited group whose members, in alphabetical order [in Greek], were the undersigned, the eminent psychiatrist Geōrgios Zavitzianos, and the distinguished professor of psychiatry Dēmētrios Kouretas. But Marie Bonaparte's support was not just limited to moral encouragement alone. She provided active and concrete assistance through her luminous guidance, her wise counsel, and her direct and invaluable collaboration. Amongst other things, she ensured that the Greek group received recognition not only in Greece, but also abroad.

As evidenced by the foregoing, Marie Bonaparte was not simply one of those great intellectual personas who work solely in the serenity of their studies. She was also a remarkable and tireless woman of action, who engaged fearlessly in all aspects of daily life. She possessed, to a truly astonishing degree, the true Bonaparte ability to effectively attend to many pursuits simultaneously. She wrote both literary and scientific works, kept abreast of scientific advances, loved the arts, made many important contributions at the major psychoanalytic conferences, and showed deep concerns for all social issues. She followed political developments attentively, was involved in numerous philanthropic institutions, and carried out many charitable works. She personally managed her household, was a devoted wife and brilliant mother, never neglected her courtly duties, and participated in all the private and public functions of the Greek royal family.

Her philanthropic work, both in times of war and peace, was truly admirable. During the Balkan Wars, she rendered invaluable services to the Hellenic Red Cross, nursing the wounded far from Athens. During the First World War, she offered similar services to the fighting French army. In times of peace, she demonstrated profound concern for all aspects of social welfare, frequently proposing significant reforms and regularly visiting numerous institutions. She was always ready to devote large sums from her considerable paternal inheritance to these causes.

Nevertheless, despite her numerous philanthropic acts, Marie Bonaparte's concern for others—and indeed her entire activity—was never confined within the bounds of conventional or formal charity. Her concern was always comprehensive and profound, and it was from this concern that all of her actions flowed: actions that were far more humanitarian, in the fullest sense of the term, than merely philanthropic. Indeed, one might add that they were deeply cultural in nature.

Amongst the many events that could—or indeed do—lend vivid relief to this remark, the following stand out in particular.

When the Caryl Chessman case was shaking the United States and the world at large, Marie Bonaparte, as might be expected, also took an interest. However, she did not limit herself to studying the case based solely on what was being said and written about the condemned man. Despite her advanced age, she travelled to the United States with the express purpose of coming into personal contact with Chessman, who had been sentenced to death, and requested the authorities to allow her to meet with him. After considerable difficulty and numerous interventions, Marie Bonaparte was eventually granted permission and held a lengthy conversation with the condemned man in prison, so that she might form her own direct and well-founded opinion of both the individual and his actions.

The Princess showed the same depth of concern in the case of Nita Baker. When this American woman, who had murdered her children at Hellēnikon, was being examined to determine the extent of her psychopathology, Marie Bonaparte—upon learning of the tragedy—did not content herself with secondhand accounts of the horrific crime. Instead, she personally visited the murderess and conducted a six-hour examination of her. As in the Chessman case, her aim was to ensure that her conclusions would be well-founded and not speculative or detached from direct observation.

Princess Marie, who was planning to write a major study—a comprehensive treatise—on the themes of criminality and justice from philosophical, psychological, and sociological perspectives, had gathered and examined an enormous number of diverse cases drawn from the domains of psychopathology and the legal system. It was with this aim in mind that she approached the two condemned individuals mentioned above, intending to include in her research materials her own personal, firsthand observations of their cases.

Marie Bonaparte's work is vast and multifaceted. It comprises purely literary works of imagination, essays and memoirs, original studies, as well as numerous translations of various writings by Freud.

In addition to the Princess' published works, there are other writings of hers that have yet to be published. It should be noted here that Marie Bonaparte intended, among other projects, to write a major study entitled "The Symbolisms of Death in Various Eras and Countries," which I do not know if she ever completed.

There also exists an extensive analytic study of the contents of five notebooks from Marie Bonaparte's childhood. To each of these notebooks corresponds a large volume she authored, in which she meticulously analyzes her childhood writings and early experiences. This substantial work, however, was never commercially published.

The study published in this issue of *Epochēs*, translated by Mrs. Liza Petridē, is an earlier psychoanalytic paper by Marie Bonaparte. Though brief, it serves as a fine example of the incisiveness and intellectual power of her mind.

For those who wish to delve further into the multifaceted and monumental oeuvre of Marie Bonaparte, a brief bibliography follows.

- *Guerres militaires et guerres sociales*, Paris, Flammarion, 1920.
- *Le Printemps sur mon jardin*, Paris, Flammarion, 1924.
- *Edgar Poe, Étude psychanalytique* (2 volumes), Paris, Denoël et Steele, 1933.
- *Topsy, Chow-Chow au poil d'or*, Paris, Denoël et Steele, 1937.
- *La Mer et le rivage*, Paris, self-published, 1940.
- *Mythes de guerre*, Imago Publishing Co., 1946.
- *Les Glanes des jours*, Imago Publishing Co., 1950.
- *Chronos, Eros et Thanatos*, Imago Publishing Co., 1951.
- *Monologues devant la Vie et la Mort*, Imago Publishing Co., 1951.
- *Les Glauques aventures de Flyda des mers*, Imago Publishing Co., 1950.
- *De la sexualité de la femme*, Paris, P.U.F., 1951.
- *Introduction à la théorie des instincts: De la prophylaxie infantile des névroses*, Paris, P.U.F., 1952.
- *Psychanalyse et biologie*, Paris, P.U.F., 1952.
- *Psychanalyse et anthropologie*, Paris, P.U.F., 1952.
- *Edgar Poe, sa vie, son oeuvre: Étude analytique*, prologue by S. Freud (3 volumes), Paris, P.U.F., 1958.

Translations of Freud's Works into French

- *Un souvenir d'enfance de Léonard de Vinci*, Paris, Gallimard, 1928.
- *Ma vie et la psychanalyse*, Paris, Gallimard, 1930.
- *Le mot d'esprit et ses rapports avec l'inconscient* (in collaboration with Dr. Marcel Nathan), Paris, Gallimard, 1930.
- *Délire et rêves dans un ouvrage littéraire: La Gradiva de Jensen*, Paris, Gallimard, 1931.
- *L'Avenir d'une illusion*, Paris, Denoël et Stele, 1932.
- *Essais de psychanalyse appliquée* (in collaboration with Mme. Edouard Marty), Paris, Denoël et Steele, 1935.
- *Cinq psychanalyses* (in collaboration with Dr. Rudolph M. Loewenstein), Paris, Denoël et Steele, 1935.
- *Métapsychologie* (in collaboration with Anne Berman), Paris, Gallimard, 1940.
- *Contributions à la psychologie de la vie amoureuse* (in collaboration with Anne Berman), *Revue française de psychanalyse, IX*, 2–21, 1936.

Besides these books, Marie Bonaparte also wrote four or five volumes of memoirs. Of these, only two have been published in a private edition under the general title *À la Mémoire des Disparus*. She also authored numerous psychoanalytic articles, studies, and presentations, several of which were published over time in the *Revue Française de Psychanalyse*, as well as in other journals.

Note

1 Editor's note: The present text was written as the introduction to the Greek edition of Marie Bonaparte's study *A Daughter's Identification with Her Dead Mother*, in a translation by Aiza Petridis, first published in *Epochēs* nos. 6, 7, and 8 (October–December 1963), and later as a monograph by Agra in 1984. Here, we are publishing the handwritten text by Andreas Embiricos, which presents several differences from the text published in *Epochēs* in 1963. Mr. Giorgēs Giatromanōlakēs contributed to the study of the handwritten text.

Chapter 6

"I Am Fighting for the Liberation of Eros"

Interview With Andreas Embiricos, Paris, January 1967

Andromachē Skarpalezou

At that time, as part of my postgraduate studies, I was working on Greek surrealism. I was doing my research in libraries and in books, that is to say using whatever had been published up to that point from the early period of Greek surrealism, namely poetry and only a few theoretical texts—statements of the movement, written, if I recall correctly, exclusively by Odysseas Elytis. In any case, I had decided to limit my personal study to these. And yet, the reputation of the surrealists, Kalamaris, Embiricos, Elytis, Engonopoulos, far outstripped what they had managed to publish. So, I thought I would add a chapter that would consist of contemporary interviews in which the spokesmen of the movement themselves would speak about whatever part of their personal experience they wished to share. The following text comes from the notes that I took during my first, and indeed only, interview with Andreas Embiricos. Within quotation marks are his words as best as I was able to record them.

"My spiritual baptism took place through Leo Tolstoy. He moved me deeply. I was a Tolstoyan. A person who felt with emotion as he thought. I was a child then, lively, sensitive, and very partial to sensual pleasures. I recognized in Tolstoy not only an artist, but also a philosopher who was fighting for what he believed was the correct worldview. From a very early age, I began to reject social falsehood and injustice, and all the evils that accumulate in the name of inhuman and artificial ideas. I tried to apply in my own life all that Tolstoy himself sought to do, renouncing the wealth of my father, who was among the richest of men. Yet despite my love for Tolstoy and my agreement with the essence of his worldview, I struggled greatly to accept and live by his teachings on Eros. I could not bear to renounce the pleasures of carnal love, nor could I forsake the enchantment of poetry. I could not separate these things from life itself. I still hold all my affection for grandfather Tolstoy, but instead of becoming a monk, I became an unbounded champion of Eros. Leo Tolstoy, like Jesus, was mistaken on this point, for if Eros and poetry are removed from life, everything else falls apart."

In my notes, I find written: Hypsikaminos [Blast Furnace], *"Roses at the Window." His reminiscences had brought this poem of his to my mind. I reproduce it here. It can be found on page 49 of the "Galaxia" edition.*

Roses at the Window

The purpose of our life is not abjection. There are things infinitely more beautiful even than that statuesque presence of the bygone epic. The purpose of our life is love. The purpose of our life is our infinite mass. The purpose of our life is to acquiesce to life itself and every one of our desires, in every place, at every moment, in every fervent stirring of what exists. The purpose of our life is the marked fleece of our existence.

"From 1921 to 1925, I lived in England, where I worked in the family business. In 1925, I went to France. I was deeply interested in psychoanalysis, and at that time I had decided to become a psychoanalyst. I underwent analysis for three years with René Laforgue and formed connections with many French psychoanalysts. Among them was Frois-Wittmann, who was also greatly interested in modern poetry. He told me he knew Breton, and I was dying to meet him. We went to see him two days later. I met a divinely inspired being. I felt the way an ancient Greek might have felt upon meeting Apollo. Not immediately, but after I returned from a trip that I had to take at that time, our meetings became regular. It was another world. I was communicating beyond the horizon, with the universality of the cosmos. The non-existence of the horizons as a barrier was being realized—the barrier created by the earth's curvature—and it was as though we were partaking in all of this in depth, height, and breadth. Every day, on the Place Blanche. Tanguy, Péret, Éluard. Personally, I had a special rapport and bond with Breton. On the Place Blanche, we would meet and talk about the surrealist movement, the group's ideas, their dissemination, the means of liberating each of us, and humankind in general, from social falsehood and injustice. We discussed Hegel, Marx, Engels, Freud.

"In earlier years, I had fully embraced Marxism. I was deeply moved by the Russian Revolution, it was in my blood, for my maternal grandmother was Russian, and a quarter of my blood is Russian. I later renounced Marxism, for it became evident in Russia that the liberation of the world cannot be achieved solely through class struggle and the proletariat. Every person must fight and undermine the foundation of the so-called 'well-established order.' One must seek absolute freedom—in thought and in life. Marxism, from the moment it became a state doctrine, resolved to enclose the spirit within narrow political criteria and interests. Directives, no matter their source, are for servile persons who accept commands contrary to the freedom of thought and, I repeat, to life. I have never accepted any conservative stance or commitment to the lifeless forms that others mistake for ideals. I desire a completely free society, much closer to liberalism than to the economism or opportunism of imperalist Marxism. A society in which each individual participates in the collective. In other words, I believe in individual liberation, which will one day lead to universal liberation. The axis of our life is Eros, whatever the present or the hoped-for society may be. And it is the most repressed condition of all, far more than any other. Surrealism and psychoanalysis have given us the means of freeing ourselves from oppressive and conventional relationships. I am a free spirit, an advocate of absolute freedom.

"In 1931, I returned to Greece, where I worked in one of my family's businesses, in a shipyard. In 1935, I resigned from my position there as director. Shortly before, strikes had taken place, and I found myself in a difficult position: on the one hand, I did not wish to appear inconsistent with my principles, yet on the other, I did not want to displease my father, toward whom I felt great gratitude. I resigned and devoted myself entirely to literature and psychoanalysis.

"We had formed a small circle of friends, Elytis, Kalamaris, and a little later Engonopoulos. Kalamaris and I, as surrealists, wanted to publish a journal of our own, so as not to cooperate with traditional publications. We wanted to call it *Ho Thiasos* [*The Troupe*]. It never came to be. Much later, I cooperated with *Nea Grammata* [*New Letters*]. In 1935, I gave the first lecture on Surrealism at the Artists' Club, the *Atelier*, on Karagiōrgē tēs Servias Street. An initiation, an introduction. It lasted over an hour. The *Atelier* had advertised it in the press. Around 150 to 200 people attended. Only a few understood, most were against it. Katsimpalēs was opposed; Karantōnēs was cautious. About 80% of the audience was deeply hostile. *Blast Furnace* had been printed in 250 copies; it sold out, not because of interest but because it was considered a scandalous book written by a madman. People quoted lines from it to mock or ridicule the author. Malice was everywhere. They mocked both the poet and the poem, as well as the entire movement. In order to set me apart from others named Embiricos, some even called me the 'Blast Furnace.' I organized an exposition of surrealist art in my home, and there, the Greek public came into contact for the first time with the works of Max Ernst, Tanguy, Magritte, Dalí, and Fernández.

"Until 1939, I made frequent trips to France, nearly every year, in order to meet with my surrealist friends. In 1941, I enlisted in the army for the Albanian campaign. Only for two months. Then the German occupation came. I did not leave Greece again until 1948.

"I devoted myself to psychoanalysis and literature. The Greek group of psychoanalysts, Kouretas, Zavitzianos, and I, could not become a component society of the IPA because of our small number of members. Our study group was formed under the aegis of the French Psychoanalytic Society. I practiced psychoanalysis for fifteen years. Afterward, I dedicated myself exclusively to literature."

The question of Andreas Embiricos' definitive cessation of his analytic practice remained obscure to me for quite some time. Much later, I learned that he had been violently and abruptly banned from practicing. I regret not having asked him about it at the time. We would then have had his personal testimony concerning an event that deserves to be considered from more than one perspective. I now continue the transcription of my notes.

"Many of my writings have not been published. Because of how libertine they are. They offend polite ears. My novel, *Ho Megas Anatolikos* [*The Great Eastern*] takes as its subject the maiden voyage of the eponymous ocean liner from England to America. Beyond the protagonists, the ship itself is symbolically a character in the work. I wrote it between 1945 and 1951. Now, I am working on my novel *Hē Polis* [*The City*]. It is Athens, although it is not named. The city itself is the subject of the work, together with the various human elements that compose it. I repeat to you: I am fighting for an absolute freedom of thought and life. For the liberation of Eros."

On his desk, I remember, there were three framed photographs: Leo Tolstoy, André Breton, and Sigmund Freud.

And there was that distinctive tone of his voice—a priestly poet, Byzantine—and the passion for storytelling, of places and times, of the course of his thought and his action. Seated on the pale-colored sofa.

Chapter 7

Psychoanalytic Glossary

Among the poet's papers was found this glossary of French psychoanalytic terms, translated into Greek, with some cross-referenced to their German equivalents (in parentheses). It is evidently A. Embiricos' personal set of notes; we decided to publish them here as supplementary material illustrating his engagement with psychoanalysis.[1]

abréaction [abreaction] (*Abreaktion*), ἐπαντίδρασις, ἐπαναντίδρασις
actif [active] (*aktiv*), ἐνεργητικὸς
amour [love] (*Liebe*), ἔρως
ambivalence (*Ambivalenz*), ἀμφιθυμία
ambivalent (*ambivalent*), ἀμφιθυμικὸς
angoisse [anxiety] (*Angst*), ἄγχος
anus (*Anus*), πρωκτὸς

bisexualité [bisexuality] (*Bisexualität*), διφυλία
bisexuel [bisexual] (*Bisexuell*), δίφυλος, διγενὴς

Ça [Id] (*Das Es*), τὸ ἐκεῖνο
captativité [captation], συλληπτικότης
censure (*Zensur*), ἔλεγχος, λογοκρισία
castration (*Kastration*), εὐνουχισμὸς
clitoris (*Klitoris*), κλειτορὶς
compensation, ἀντισταθμιστικὸν ἀντάλλαγμα
coït (*Coitus*), συνουσία
conscient [conscious] (*bewußt*) συνειδητὸς
conflit [conflict] (*Konflikt*), διαμάχη
conversion (*Konversion*), σωματικοποίησις, μεταλλοτροπία, ἀλλοτροπία
condensation (*Verdichtung*), συμπύκνωσις
complexe [complex] (*Komplex*), σύμπλεγμα
complexualité [complexuality], συμπλεγματικότης
cunnilingus, αἰδοιολειχία
culpabilité [guilt] (*Schuld, Schuldbewußtsein*), ἐνοχὴ

déplacement [displacement] (*Verschiebung*), μετατόπισις
déplaisir [unpleasure] (*Unlust*), ἀφηδονισμὸς
défoulement [discharge], ἐξαπώθησις
déflorer [to deflower], διακορεύω, διαπαρθενεύω
défloration [deflowering], διακόρευσις, διαπαρθένευσις
déterminism [determinism] (*Determinismus*), ντετερμινισμός, προσδιορισμὸς
dynamisme [dynamism] (*Dynamismus*), δυναμισμὸς
dynamique [dynamic] (*dynamisch*), δυναμικὸς

éjaculation [ejaculation] (*Ejakulation*), ἐκσπερμάτωσις
éjaculer [to ejaculate] (*Ejakulieren*), ἐκσπερματώνω, ἐκσπερματίζω
élaboration [elaboration/working-through], ἐπεξεργασία
érection [erection] (*Erektion*), στύσις
éros (*Eros*), ἔρως
érotisme [eroticism] (*Erotismus*), ἐρωτισμὸς
érotisme oral [oral eroticism] (*oraler Erotismus*), στοματικὸς ἐρωτισμὸς
érotisme anal (*analer Erotismus*), πρωκτικὸς ἐρωτισμὸς
érotisme génital (*genitaler Erotismus*), γεννητικὸς ἐρωτισμὸς
exhibitionnnisme (exhibitionism) (*Schaulust*), ἐκθετισμὸς
exhibitionniste (exhibitionist), ἐκθέτης, -ου, ἐκθέτις, -ιδος
excrément (excrement/feces) (*Kot*), περίττωμα

fixation (*Fixierung*), ἐνσφήνωσις
femme phallique [phallic woman] (*phallische Frau*), πεοφόρος γυνὴ
fellatio (*Fellatio*), πεολειχία
frigidité [frigidity] (*Frigidität*), δυσπαρευνία
feminité [feminity] (*Weiblichkeit*), θηλύτης, θηλυκότης

génital (*genital*), γεννητικὸς
genitalité [genitality] (*Genitalität*), γεννητικότης

hétérosexuel (*heterosexuell*), φιλετερόφυλος
hétérosexualité (*Heterosexualität*), φιλετεροφυλία
homosexuel (*homosexuell*), φιλομόφυλος
homosexualité (*Homosexualität*), φιλομοφυλία

inconscient (unconscious) (*unbewußt*, *Unbewußtsein*), ἀσυνείδητον
introjection (*Introjektion*), ἐνδοβολὴ
introversion (*Introverzion*), ἐνδοστροφὴ
introverti [introvert(ed)], ἐνδόστροφος
invertion [inversion], ἀναστροφὴ
inverti [invert(ed)], ἀνάστροφος
impulsion [impulse] (*Impuls*), παρόρμησις

instinct (*Instinkt*, *Trieb*), ὁρμέμφυτον, ἔνστικτον
impuissance [impotence] (*Impotenz*), ἀνικανότης

libido (*Libido*), λιβιδὼ
loi du talion [*lex talionis*], νόμος τοῦ ἀντιπεπονθότος
latence [latency] (*Latenz*), λανθία, λανθανότης

moi [ego] (*Ich*), ἐγὼ
masturbation (*Masturbation*, *Onanismus*), αὐνανισμὸς
masturbation clitoridienne [clitoral masturbation], κλειτορικὸς ἢ κλειτοριδικὸς αὐνανισμὸς
masturbation vaginale [vaginal masturbation], αὐνανισμὸς τοῦ κόλπου
masturbation uréthrale [urethral masturbation], οὐρηθρικὸς αὐνανισμὸς
masturbation anale [anal masturbation], πρωκτικὸς αὐνανισμὸς

narcissisme [narcissism] (*Narzissismus*), ναρκισσισμὸς
narcissique [narcissistic] (*narzissistisch*), ναρκισσευτικὸς
négation [negation] (*Verneinung*), ἄρνησις
négation de la réalité [negation of reality] (*Realitätsverneinung*), ἄρνησις τῆς πραγματικότητος

orgasme [orgasm] (*Orgasmus*), ὀργασμὸς

psychanalyse [psychoanalysis] (*Psychoanalyse*), ψυχοανάλυσις
plaisir [pleasure] (*Lust*), ἡδονὴ
pénis (*Penis*), πέος
principe du plaisir [pleasure principle] (*Lustprinzip*), ἀρχὴ τῆς ἡδονῆς
principe de réalité [reality principle] (*Realitätsprinzip*), ἀρχὴ τῆς πραγματικότητος
Phallus (*Phallus*), φαλλὸς
préconscient [preconscious] (*vorbewußt*, *Vorbewußtsein*), προ-συνειδητὸν
projection (*Projektion*), προβολὴ
pulsion [drive] (*Trieb*), ὦσις
puissance [potency] (*Potenz*), ἱκανότης
psychisme [mental apparatus/psychic life] (*Psychismus*), ψυχισμὸς
psychose [psychosis] (*Psychose*), ψύχωσις
psychonévrose [psychoneurosis] (*Psychonevrose*), ψυχονεύρωσις
phantasme [phantasy] (*Phantasie*), φαντασίωσις
puberté [puberty] (*Pubertät*), ἥβη, ἐφηβεία
prégénital [pregenital] (*Prägenital*), προγεννητικὸς
préœdipien [pre-Oedipal] (*Präödipal*), προοιδιποδικός, προοιδιποδικὸν
punition [punishment] (*Strafe*, *Strafbedürfnis*), τιμωρία
potentiel [potential], δυναμικὸν

refoulement [repression] (*Verdrängnung*), ἀπώθησις
refouler [to repress] (*verdrängen*), ἀπωθῶ
rationalisation (*Rationalisierung*), ἐκλογίκευσις
réalité [reality] (*Realität*), πραγματικότης
rendre conscient [to make conscious] (*bewußtmachen*), συνειδητοποιῶ
résistance (*Wiederstand*), ἀντίστασις

sperme [sperm] (*Sperma*), σπέρμα
sexe [sex/gender] (*Geschlecht*), φῦλον
sexualité [sexuation] (*Sexualität*), φυλετικότης
sadisme [sadism] (*Sadismus*), σαδισμὸς
surmoi [superego] (*Überich*), ὑπερεγὼ
sublimation (*Sublimieren*), μετουσίωσις, ἐξύψωσις
sodomiser [to sodomize], σοδομίζω
sodomie [sodomy], σοδομισμὸς
substitut [substitute] (*Ersatz*), ὑποκατάστατον

tabou [taboo] (*Tabu*), ταμπού
traumatisme (*Trauma*), τραυματισμὸς
toute-puissance [omnipotence] (*Allmacht*), παντοδυναμία
toute-puissance anale [anal omnipotence], πρωκτικὴ παντοδυναμία
toute-puissance de la pensée [omnipotence of thoughts] (*Allmacht der Gedenken*), παντοδυναμία τῆς σκέψεως

vagin (*Vagina*), κόλπος
vulve [vulva], αἰδοῖον
voyeurisme [voyeurism] (*Schaulust*), ὀπταστισμὸς
voyeur, ὀπταστὴς

zones érogènes [erogenous zones] (*erogene Zonen*), ἐρωτογόνοι ζῶναι

Note

1 Translator's note: English translations from the French in brackets have been added where necessary.

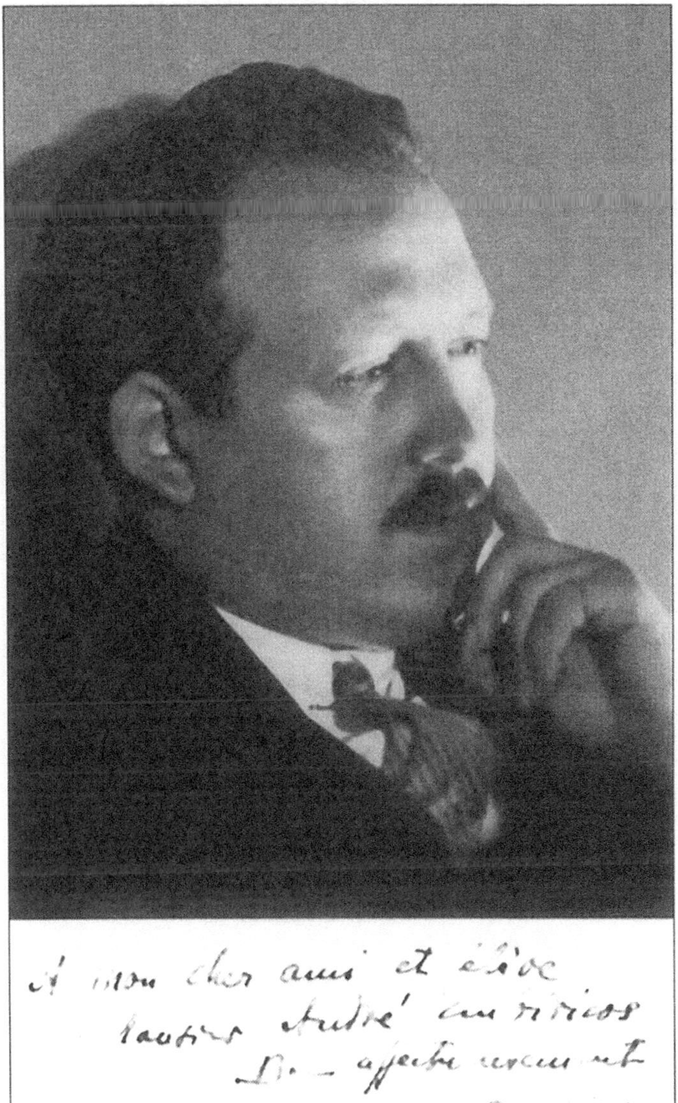

Figure 7.1 Photograph of René Laforgue with a handwritten dedication to Andreas Embiricos.

Part II

Critical Essays on Embiricos as Analyst

Chapter 8

Andreas Embiricos' Overseas Journey and Psychoanalytic Circumnavigations

Thanasēs Tzavaras

Andreas Embiricos traversed the twentieth century in an active, cosmopolitan, and at times dilettantish manner. The celebratory atmosphere surrounding the centenary of his birth could be regarded as an extremely Surrealist gesture, one that Greek society now offers him in recompense, after decades of scorn and erratic rumor-mongering. I am of course aware that, despite the singular approach he took towards the publication of his poetic work, both specialists and, more broadly, the educated Greek public have come to recognize the importance of his work and to delight in the pleasures his creations afford. His biographical details are already well known and will be further illuminated by the commemorative events. In this way, the transoceanic voyage of this cosmopolitan and patrician creator will come even more fully into view.[1]

In the following text, an attempt will be made to more precisely identify the key points, anchorages, and tempests of his psychoanalytic voyage—elements which, in my view, remain relatively unknown. The publication in the present volume of the only two psychoanalytic texts known until recently by Andreas Embiricos the analyst, along with the additional presentation here of a newly discovered text—that of a lecture given by Embiricos himself—allows for a more complete picture of Embiricos the pioneering, first-in-his-class Greek psychoanalyst.[2]

The table at the end of this chapter provides an overview of the political and psychoanalytic events that punctuated and characterized Andreas Embiricos' circumnavigation of the psychoanalytic continent. As I have written elsewhere, psychoanalytic ideas and a few psychoanalytic texts had already begun to circulate in pre-war Greece, and a certain critical discourse had already emerged in the country by that time. Allow me to remind the reader that this circulation of ideas was chiefly due to the work of a few progressive intellectuals, mainly academics. The important role played by linguist Manolis Triandaphyllidēs and the members of the Educational Club in the transmission and dissemination of psychoanalytic ideas in pre-war Greece has long been known, as has the almost unanimous opposition to psychoanalytic ideas not only by the University's philosophical and medical establishment, but also by non-academic circles. Lastly, it will be unnecessary to emphasize how inimical religious and ecclesiastical milieus were towards Freud's theories.

Andreas Embiricos obviously did not directly take part in this early movement, as he was only in his 20s at the time, although he was aware of it. We know he enrolled in the Philosophical School in 1919, yet no written traces that we know of survive that might substantiate any such information. Instead, his background, his failed attempts at participating in his family's business, and his cosmopolitan nature all prompted him to leave Greece for Western Europe, which was then undergoing a renaissance in the wake of the devastation of the First World War. During his life abroad from 1925 to 1931, in London, Paris, and other Western capitals, he encountered psychoanalysis mainly through the importance the French Surrealists accorded it and the way in which they engaged with it. We know that the young Andreas Embiricos met Breton in 1927 and that his enthusiasm about their encounter was a decisive factor in his subsequent artistic and psychoanalytic choices.

French society at that time was characterized by its traditional anti-German attitude and was often dominated by generalized racism and anti-Semitism. It was still licking its wounds after the carnage of the First World War and had not forgotten its humiliating 1897 defeat in the Franco-German War. It had the utmost difficulty accepting anything German, and so it was natural that Freudian ideas were introduced with a great deal of delay. The Paris Psychoanalytic Society was founded only in 1926, and from the start, two tendencies appeared within its ranks: one internationalist, advocating for the universal significance of psychoanalytic ideas and their applications; the other Franco-centric, which for a considerable time sought to establish a distinctly French psychoanalysis, purged of all German or Jewish elements. This conflict would, in effect, persist until the Second World War and perhaps even beyond it—that is, until the reopening of the Psychoanalytic Institute in Paris following the German occupation.

By way of example, I now present two brief excerpts that shed light on the prevailing intellectual atmosphere of the 1920s and 1930s. The first is a polemical comment: "*Psychanarchy* is like the dictatorship of the neural proletariat over the higher psychic functions, which under normal conditions ought to maintain control over it." And yet another text from the same atmosphere of reactionary mass literature. We read, from the pen of a certain "Noge," the following charming lines (charming, that is, for that era):

> Here, we have before us a legendary figure of modern literature, Freud, prepared and heralded by Bergson, Dostoyevski, Proust and Einstein. Thanks to this Messiah, who sails aboard the good ship *Libido*, all devourers of dreams may voyage across the ocean of sexuality, until they reach the Gulf of Incest, where the Golden Fleece of the Oedipus Complex is bestowed.[3]

It was within this atmosphere that Andreas Embiricos gravitated towards psychoanalysis and began an analysis with René Laforgue, the Alsatian founder of the Paris Psychoanalytic Society. Here, it is useful to provide some information about René Laforgue (1894–1962). Born in Alsace under German rule, the German-speaking Laforgue became the first French psychoanalyst, thanks to his bilingualism, and attempted an initial reconciliation of German psychoanalysis with "*l'esprit français*." He settled in Paris in 1922 and was analyzed by Eugénie Sokolnicka, a Polish Jew who had been living in Paris since 1904. Sokolnicka, who had a degree in the sciences, was also a writer and the analyst of many well-known French psychoanalysts and artists, including André Gide. Despite her many professional successes, she was marginalized both because of her origins and because she was not a medical doctor. She eventually committed suicide in 1934. In 1923, Laforgue began an important correspondence with Freud that lasted until 1937. These letters contain a great deal of information concerning the foundation of the Paris Psychoanalytic Society, the *Revue Française de Psychanalyse*, and the *Évolution Psychiatrique* group.

Although Laforgue was the founder of French psychoanalysis, once Princess Marie Bonaparte became involved in psychoanalytic affairs with the support of Polish-Jewish psychiatrist Rudolph Loewenstein, who had moved from Berlin to Paris in 1925, Laforgue lost the presidency, which had an effect on his postwar fate. A man caught between two cultures and languages, with no clear internationalist tendencies like those mentioned previously, he became involved in a political misadventure that cost him both his reputation and his disciples. Laforgue had attempted, albeit ambivalently, to gain some advantage from the German occupiers through his correspondence with the infamous Matthias Heinrich Göring, the gravedigger of Freudian psychoanalysis in Hitler's Germany, in the hope of somehow carving out a politically acceptable and purely French psychoanalysis from internationalist and Jewish-dominated Freudian psychoanalysis. After the war, he would be accused of collaborating with the occupier and, although he was acquitted for lack of evidence (which would come to light years after his death), he nonetheless had fallen into disrepute and was marginalized. He ended his career surrounded by some of his students at his final residence in Casablanca.

One of the protagonists of the reaction against Laforgue was Marie Bonaparte, who, despite her royal lineage, was a fanatical opponent of the German and Nazi state. Laforgue's analysts and disciples encountered various difficulties being recognized in the postwar psychoanalytic environment of Paris. Apart from Embiricos, amongst them were two other Greeks involved in psychoanalysis: Froso Karapanou and Nikolaos Drakoulidēs, who claimed to be Laforgue's friend. Although Andreas Embiricos continued to see Laforgue regularly through his last pre-war trip abroad and referred Froso Karapanou to him for a second analysis in Paris after the war, he seems not to have maintained close contact with his former analyst after that time. Instead, following Marie Bonaparte's return to Greece in 1946 and the creation of the first psychoanalytic study group, the princess and the poet became close friends.

It will be useful to recall here—as evidenced by their correspondence, which I have previously commented on[4]—that they shared a deep concern over the possibility of a Third World War, this time nuclear in nature. Indeed, they even considered settling together in Florida in the United States, a region they presumed outside the theater of war and whose climate was reminiscent of Greece's. It should also be recalled that in this fantasied move abroad, Andreas Embiricos planned on playing the role of secretary to Marie Bonaparte. Regardless of any such plans, however, it should be stressed here that Andreas Embiricos had great respect for Marie Bonaparte and her work. This is demonstrated by his preface to her *Latent Necrophilia in the Work of Edgar Poe* (1944); his translation of the Princess' three lectures at Parnassus, published by the Hellenic Psychoanalytic Group in 1950 (recently brought to light through the discovery of relevant manuscripts by Embiricos); his biographical preface to "Identification of a Girl with Her Dead Mother" in *Epochēs* (1963); and especially his dithyrambic 1963 biographical piece, published here for the first time.

But let us return to 1935, when, against the backdrop of the total rejection of Surrealism and scorn for psychoanalysis by the conservative Greek intelligentsia, and amidst the unprecedented social and political turmoil of 1930s Greece, Embiricos decided to publicly identify himself as a Surrealist poet with the publication of *Blast Furnace* and to enter private practice as a psychoanalyst. It should be remembered that in the 1930s, the only services offered in Greece and Athens for the mentally ill were both few and archaic. Apart from asylums and private clinics, the only type of talk therapy offered was through "counseling stations" that Dimitrios Moraitis had sponsored, inspired by Adlerian psychology. Several keen psychiatrists, such as Dimitrios Kouretas, or educators, such as Manolis Triantaphyllidēs, took part in this first psychotherapeutic offering aimed mainly at children and their parents. Georgios Zavitzianos, a psychiatrist who also returned from France at the end of the 1930s, had similar interests. The only person providing formal psychoanalysis of adult neurotics was therefore Andreas Embiricos, who, as far as we can tell, had no interactions with any other specialist in Greece, though he maintained ongoing contact with Laforgue and other French psychoanalysts.[5]

In 1940, the war interrupted all communication between Embiricos and his contacts in Western Europe, including with the relevant literature. He remained in constant contact with a close circle of intellectuals and artists, and in 1940 he married his first wife, Matsi Chatzilazarou, a highly interesting poet and former analysand of his (it is worth noting in passing that René Laforgue, his own analyst, had also taken as his second wife a former analysand, Délia Clauzel). The global psychoanalytic movement witnessed many such marriages and, as such, this was not considered an unusual practice provided, of course, that rules separating the therapeutic relationship from the private one had been observed. Naturally, such a decision cannot be regarded merely as a matter of psychodynamic technique. In any case, this subject is not one of the more illustrious chapters in the history of psychoanalysis.[6]

Their marriage did not last beyond the end of the German occupation, when Matsi Chatzilazarou left for Paris, where she frequented the circles of Greek intellectuals in exile there. In January 1947, Andreas Embiricos married Vivika Zisi, with his close friend Odysseus Elytis as his best man.

Following the episode during which Embiricos was taken hostage by the Greek paramilitary Communist organization "OPLA" (an event that has been studied by specialists) and after the restoration of the monarchy in 1946, a psychoanalytic study group began to form around Marie Bonaparte, including psychiatrists Georgios Zavitzianos and Dimitrios Kouretas as its main participants. Regular meetings involving psychoanalytic discussions and clinical supervision took place at Marie Bonaparte's home in Athens, at the corner of Akademias and Lycabettus Streets. As has long been documented by historical research, these meetings were attended by various intellectuals, as is also attested by Georgios Theotokas. Alongside his participation in this group, Embiricos continued to see patients in his private practice, which he had not interrupted during the German occupation. In his capacity as a training analyst, he also undertook the analysis of the aforementioned psychiatrists Georgios Zavitzianos and Dimitrios Kouretas. This first nucleus of psychoanalysts in Athens was favorably received by the Paris Psychoanalytic Society under the patronage of Marie Bonaparte and with the agreement of Ernest Jones and Anna Freud, who, moreover, made an official visit to Athens in January 1949.[7]

In 1950, the three Greek psychoanalysts were admitted as members of the Paris Psychoanalytic Society. As a prerequisite for membership, each published a case study in the *Revue Française de Psychanalyse* that same year. Embiricos' case study is reproduced in the present volume.

We should again recall that the 1940s were extremely difficult years for everyone in Greece; the three psychoanalysts, too, encountered great difficulties in their daily professional lives, which included being able to earn a living and to maintain their contacts with the international psychoanalytic community and its literature. Moreover, the academic establishment had not softened its opposition to psychoanalysis, and various actions had begun to be taken to counter the nascent attempts at the institutionalization of psychoanalysis in Greece. We should take this context into account in attempting to understand Georgios Zavitzianos' almost forced emigration to North America for economic reasons, as well as Froso Karapanou's earlier departure from Greece to pursue higher education. The reasons behind the rumors regarding Andreas Embiricos' falling afoul of the police should also be sought in the sinister climate of this period. An unsubstantiated rumor exists within the collective memory of the Greek psychoanalytic community that he was supposedly forced to shut down his practice by official decree. However, archival research has failed to uncover any concrete event that would substantiate such a rumor, and both his relatives and our mutual acquaintances have assured us of the contrary. It nonetheless remains possible, as Dimitrios Kouretas once remarked to us, that someone may have "ratted him out" and that he was subsequently harassed by an arbitrary authority. But the allegation that a patient of his committed suicide while in treatment with him and such like all belong to the murky memories of a turbulent era. Moreover, it should be recalled that during the same period, 1949–50, the Communist intelligentsia, via an article signed by a pseudonymous "Marinos," for the first time explicitly denounced psychoanalysis as a bourgeois ideology.[8]

Be that as it may, it appears that Embiricos, disgusted by this and other things, decided to close down his practice in April 1951 and left for Paris. Around the same time, Marie Bonaparte was forced to leave for Paris to seek medical treatment for a fractured femur she had suffered during a fall at home. After participating in the International Psychoanalytic Association conference in Amsterdam, Embiricos and his wife would remain in Paris until 1953–4, when he returned to settle in Athens. Although he never again resumed clinical work, he nonetheless maintained his membership in the Paris Psychoanalytic Society until the early 1960s, but otherwise devoted himself exclusively to his artistic activities, namely writing and photography.

Until his death in 1975, according to several convergent reports, he never ceased being interested in psychoanalytic matters, mainly by keeping abreast of the psychoanalytic literature as much as possible. Indeed, according to reports from his relatives, on one of his last trips to London in 1973, Embiricos spent time in the well-known psychoanalytic bookshop Karnak, where he perused and purchased a number of recent editions and publications.

The fact remains that, apart from the sole interview he gave to Andromachē Skarpalezou in 1967 in the magazine *Ēridanos*,[9] we know of no other written or oral reference by Andreas Embiricos to his clinical work or thought. For years, only one text had been found in his papers; this is the second clinical case published in this volume. It seems that Embiricos, prolific writer that he was, did leave behind other notes or drafts on psychoanalytic topics. Recent efforts to retrieve these from his entourage have borne some fruit, and the text of one of his lecture courses, which was recently found, is also being published here. I had previously hypothesized that one could approach Embiricos' published literary texts by looking for their psychoanalytic origins and influences and, from these, one might also deduce his sources of inspiration and gather information about the type of psychoanalysis he promoted and practiced. The relatively recent and posthumous publication of *The Great Eastern* [*Megalos Anatolikos*] makes this project particularly painstaking and obviously a subject for specialist studies. In the meantime, as we await a psychoanalytic biography of Embiricos to complement the works of literary criticism written about him, we should be especially skeptical toward some of the popular critical stances taken toward him. For example, I have recently argued the case that *Zemphira or The Secret of Pasiphae* [*Zemphyra ē to mystikon tēs*

Pasiphaēs] should be approached as a highly elaborated literary version of Freud's positions in "A Child Is Being Beaten."[10]

Therefore, in light of what I have written in this chapter, the events organized in celebration of the centenary of his birth will hopefully provide the impetus for new research that will allow for a better acquaintance with Embiricos the psychoanalyst and his place in early Freudian psychoanalytic theory under the influence of those psychoanalytic themes particularly dear to the Surrealists: the automatic productions of the unconscious, the overvaluing of dreams, and, above all, the great importance these circles attached to sexual liberation as a source of salvation and liberation for mankind.

Table 8.1 Chronological Table of the Introduction of Psychoanalysis in Greece

Political Events	*Psychoanalytic Events*	*Events in the Life of Andreas Embiricos*
		1901: Birth
1902: Burglary of Tatoi Palace 1908: Cretan Revolution 1909: Goudi Coup		
1912–13: Balkan Wars	1912: Translation of an article by Th. Reik 1915: Article by M. Triantaphyllidēs on linguistics and psychoanalysis	
1916: National Schism 1917–18: First World War 1918: Greek Communist Party (KKE) founded		
1919: Southern Russia Intervention		1919: Enrolls in the Philosophical School of Athens
1919–22: War in Asia Minor 1922: Defeat—Asia Minor Catastrophe 1922: Military coup d'état		
1924: Democracy restored	1924: Introductory article in favor of psychoanalysis by I. Imvriōtēs (left-wing)	
1925: Pangalos dictatorship	1925: Translation of Freud's *Group Psychology* and *Three Essays*	1925–30: Studies in London and Paris

(*Continued*)

Table 8.1 (Continued)

Political Events	*Psychoanalytic Events*	*Events in the Life of Andreas Embiricos*
1926: Kondylis dictatorship	1926: Article in favor of psychoanalysis by K. Sōtērios (left-wing)	1926–30: Personal analysis with René Laforgue
	1927: E. Lambridēs publishes counterattack against negative criticism of psychoanalysis by philosophers	
	1928: Favorable introductory article in *Hellenic Medicine* journal	
	1928: Series of articles by M. Triantaphyllidēs introducing Adlerian psychoanalysis.	
	1931: Anti-Freud by Ch. Androustos (conservative-religious)	1931: Return to Athens
	1931–9: Series of essays and presentations by Zouranēs, Imvriōtēs, Kouretas, and Kōnstantinidēs	
	1932: First translation of Wilhelm Reich	
	1932–9: *Individual Psychology*, an Adlerian journal, founded by D. Mōraïtēs	
1933: Plastiras coup		
1935: Venizelos coup—Kondylis countercoup		1935: Starts private practice in Athens. Publishes *Blast Furnace*.
1935: Referendum—monarchy restored		
1936–41: Metaxas dictatorship		1936–9: Ongoing collegial relationship with Laforgue

(*Continued*)

Table 8.1 (Continued)

Political Events	*Psychoanalytic Events*	*Events in the Life of Andreas Embiricos*
1940: Greco-Italian War		
1941: Greco-German War		
1941–4: German, Italian, and Bulgarian occupation	1942: D. Kouretas named professor of neurology and psychiatry at University of Thessaloniki	
1944: Liberation		
1944: Dekemvriana	1944: Translation of *Necrophilia of Poe* by Marie Bonaparte	1944: Writes introduction to Marie Bonaparte's *Latent Necrophilia in the Work of Edgar Poe*
		1944–5: Kidnapped and taken hostage by OPLA
1946: Referendum—monarchy restored		
1946–9: Civil war	1946–9: Study group formed around Marie Bonaparte	
	1949: The study group becomes a member of the Société psychanalytique de Paris (SPP)	1949: Becomes a member of the SPP; takes part in the first IPA conference in Zurich
	1949–50: Papers by the Greek members published in the *RFP*	1950: Publishes a paper in the *RFP*; the Greek psychoanalytic study group publishes Embiricos' unsigned translation of Marie Bonaparte's *Three Introductory Lectures to Psychoanalysis*
	1949: Anna Freud's visit to Athens	
	1949: Marie Bonaparte gives three public lectures in Athens	
	1949–50: Strident antipsychoanalytic article published in a Marxist periodical	

(Continued)

Table 8.1 (Continued)

Political Events	*Psychoanalytic Events*	*Events in the Life of Andreas Embiricos*
	1950: G. Zavitzianos emigrates to the United States	
	c. 1951: Final departure of Marie Bonaparte from Greece	1951: Permanently retires from clinical practice; leaves for Paris; participates in the second IPA conference in Amsterdam
		1960: Radio talk with D. Kouretas and D. Myrat on psychoanalysis
	1962: Death of Marie Bonaparte	1963: Writes an introduction to Bonaparte's *Identification of a Girl with Her Dead Mother*
1967–74: Greek Junta dictatorship		
		1975: Death in Athens

Notes

1 Here, I am solely referring to the recent tributes in the daily and periodical press, pending their publication in a collected format, which will not happen in any case until after the commemorative events have finished: "Andreas Empeirikos: Pais en tē kaminō, Prosōpa—21os Aiōnas," *Ta Nea*, 27 May 2000; "Tēs mē symmorphōseōs hagios: Andreas Empeirikos 1901–1975," *Anti*, 9 February 2001; "Opheiloume na eugnōmonoume tous poiētes: 100 chronia apo tēn gennēsē tou Andrea Empeirikou," *Hē Augē*, 5 April 2001.

2 Archives are like mines, or better, like archaeological digs, to use one of Freud's favorite metaphors. You don't know exactly what you're looking for and, most importantly, you don't know what you'll end up finding. This is complicated by the fact that Embiricos followed an idiosyncratic strategy for the publication of his work. Concerning his psychoanalytic writings, we don't have enough evidence despite the existence of his sole publication in the *Revue Française de Psychanalyse*. It nonetheless seems that Embiricos wrote, or at least noted down, many things touching on psychoanalysis. While recently discovered texts or notes indicate a continued engagement with psychoanalytic matters, it remains to be determined

whether they might have been intended for publication. For an overview of the current state of research regarding Embiricos as psychoanalyst, see: Thanasēs Tzavaras, "Ho Andreas Empeirikos kai hē psychanalysē," *Deltio tēs Hetaireias Spoudōn Neoellēnikou Politismou kai Genikēs Paideias* no. 5 (1981): 80–8. See also: Thanasēs Tzavaras, "Stoicheia kai sēmeia apo dyo archeia," in *Psychanalysē kai Hellada* (Athens: Hetaireia Spoudōn Neoellēnikou Politismou kai Genikēs Paideias, 1984), 89–105; Thanasēs Tzavaras, "Ho Andreas Empeirikos kai hē psychanalysē II," *Chartes* no. 17/18 (1985): 566–76.

3 For more on the prevailing atmosphere in the crucial decades of the 1920s and 1930s, see: Élisabeth Roudinesco, *Histoire de la psychanalyse en France: La bataille de cent ans*, vol. 1 (1982), vol 2. (1986) (Paris: Seuil). See also, from a foreign perspective: Peter Gay, *Freud: A Life for Our Time* (London: J. M. Dent & Sons, 1988). For general information on this period, see: Thanasēs Tzavaras. "Ho Bergson kai hē gallikē neuropsychiatrikē paradosē," *Neusis* no. 8 (1999): 55–69, from which the aforementioned citations were drawn.

4 In the volume Thanasēs Tzavaras (ed.), *Psychanalysē kai Hellada—Stoicheia, theseis, erōtēmata* (Athens: Hetaireia Spoudōn Neoellēnikou Politismou kai Genikēs Paideias, 1984), 99–103.

5 It has recently been confirmed by Embiricos' close associates that he made an annual trip to Paris, where he met with his psychoanalyst as well as other French psychoanalysts, evidently for professional reasons. He also kept himself abreast of developments in the literature. Indirect sources indicate that he possessed an extensive psychoanalytic library which, regrettably, cannot now be assessed as the volumes appear to have been dispersed over the years and after multiple relocations.

6 According to a statement made by Matsi Chatzilazarou to the author of the present text in the early 1980s, her transition from analysand to wife occurred in full accordance with the rules of the art. This, of course, did not prevent the difficulties that arose in their marriage. These lines are written to underscore the fact that, particularly amongst first- and second generation psychoanalysts, entanglements of transference and omnipotence were not uncommon—beginning with Freud himself, who analyzed his own daughter, Anna.

7 The extant documents concerning this visit were recently published in the psychoanalytic journal *Ek tōn Hysterōn* (special issue, 1999). My assessment of such a gesture—paternalistic in nature—is entirely negative, given that psychoanalysis cannot be transmitted through visits, even of a symbolic character. It is worth underscoring that the same symptom reappeared more recently in the form of a visit by Jacques Lacan's daughter, Judith Miller.

8 The reference is to the well-known article published in *Antaios*. This is not the appropriate place for a more detailed analysis of this particular symptom of the Communist Left—especially at a moment when the defeat of the Communists in the Greek Civil War had become a certainty. In a recent brief text of mine (*He Augē*, 5 April 2001), I began to develop the idea that one of the "casualties" of the Greek Civil War might also be

considered psychoanalysis—at least insofar as it was introduced by the members of the first psychoanalytic group.

9 Published in English translation in the present volume.

10 S. Freud, "Ein Kind wird geschlagen," *Gesammelte Werke* XII (1919): 197–226. In English translation: "A Child Is Being Beaten," *S.E.* XVII, 175–204. See also Thanasēs Tzavaras, "Ho prōtos Hellēnas psychanalytēs," *Ta Nea*, 27 May 2000.

Chapter 9

A Case of Psychoanalytic Practice With Surrealistic Peregrinations[1]

Erē Kourla and Giōrgos Kourias

In 1950, three articles by Greek psychoanalysts were published in volume 14 of the *Revue française de psychanalyse*, the official journal of the French Psychoanalytic Society. This was the "God helps those who help themselves" moment by which Zavitzianos, Kouretas, and Embiricos sought to introduce their Greek psychoanalytic study group, recognized by the International Psychoanalytic Society under the aegis of the French Society. Despite their group's aristocratic patroness, their attempt proved ineffectual. These three texts are all that is left behind as written evidence of domestic psychoanalytic activity in Greece, which seems not to have been so sterile after all. The paper authored by the poet stands out amongst the three, and it will be our subject here. It is entitled "*Un cas de névrose obsessionnelle avec éjaculations précoces*" [A case of obsessional neurosis with premature ejaculations], and it is the presentation of an analytic treatment conducted by Andreas Embiricos.[2]

It would seem that in the person of Embiricos, Greek intelligentsia possesses a unique distinction on a global scale. He is regarded as the only example of a (practicing) psychoanalyst who was also a (professional) poet. Verifying this fact is not only practically impossible, but also of little significance. Unverifiable though it is, this notion, while prevalent, loses nothing of its allure. And when the poet in question is a Surrealist of the caliber of Andreas Embiricos, this allure becomes an invitation to reflection and inquiry; meanwhile, his only extant[3] psychoanalytic text seems to become a promise—one that hints at the revelation of the tender secrets underlying his art. But to the reader who will want to engage in such contemplation, no such secret will be revealed. Perhaps, like us, he will come to love Embiricos the poet even more.

One can find many affinities, as the case may be, between a literary work and a psychoanalytic text. However, they are by no means the same thing. The protagonist differs: in the second case, and only in that case, it is the unconscious itself, given that what is at stake here is the transmittal of a therapeutic process. Yet, the author remains an author, and as such he inevitably maintains, through his authorial practice, a privileged relationship with the unconscious—this time his own. If one wants to approach Embiricos' dual professional role from this perspective, then his psychoanalytic monograph together with his poetic work form a rather complex ensemble. Within this ensemble, however, certain "moments" of the author's functioning can be discerned—moments significant enough to be of interest in a possible reconsideration of the established notion that genuine literary activity cannot coexist with the practice of psychoanalysis.

This is all from the perspective of a writer-analyst. However, it is also interesting to note the corresponding role-distribution that emerges. In a clinical monograph, the one analyzed is the patient; in literature, if anyone is being analyzed, it is the reader. We ask that we be permitted this expansive use of the term, as we believe that it holds some truth.

The fact that poetry[4] and clinical psychoanalysis share the same tool—the word—despite its symptomatic façade, reveals their internal affinity, their shared, deep-rooted origin in the essence of speech: the perpetual substitution of one meaning for another, not as the consequence of the putative intent of a subject, but as the result of the structural ambiguity of the word itself. This springs from the latter's lack of any absolute identity, at its core is a metaphor:

> Speech arises from opposition. Initially, it feels the urge to say: "this is that," precisely because what initially exists is a "this is not that." It is as if the primary function of speech were the negation of a difference, and as if this negation confirmed being. In a highly paradoxical way, in and through speech, being is a negation of negation. It is not fundamentally an affirmation.[5]

Meaning is something that is constantly slipping away and eluding successive acts of signification, never anchoring itself in any of them. Following the trajectory of metaphor, its zigzagging journey opens up pathways into regions not under the direct supervision of consciousness. Might it not be the case that both psychoanalytic interpretation and poetic architectonics are taken along as passengers on this journey? And is it not in the emergence of a new way of listening that the authenticity of artistic creation is ultimately to be recognized, when the curve of the mind retrieves fragments of reality from silence? The Surrealists understood this very well. Let us recall that work by Magritte that depicts (literally) a pipe in all its naturalistic glory and fidelity, yet contains the carefully calligraphed caption—part of the painting itself, not its title—"*ceci n'est pas une pipe*." This is no mere attempt at easy sensationalism; it is the unwavering declaration of a belief, and at the same time, an invitation to the viewer for a minimal yet essential consensus, one necessary for engaging with the artist's work.

Andreas Embiricos, a painter of love, calls upon us with all of his psychic strength not to deny the play of images. Conquered by Surrealism rather than a follower of it, he made it his goal, as is well known, to seize the truth not by overcoming reality, but by penetrating deep into its secrets, breaking through it. His love of materiality and his privileging of the concrete is what his "poem-event" expresses; to achieve this, he had to plow through the entire Greek language. For this conquest of reality is its very transference into poetic creation itself; strange, accidental, and unknown relationships of the real must be incorporated into the poem's becoming. If the reader is "analyzed" while reading it, it is because poetic and psychoanalytic discourse have this in common: they are both discourses of revelation.

Behind Some Surfaces

At first glance, Embiricos' psychoanalytic writing does not resemble his literary work. Written in a sparc and measured style, it is, on the contrary, strongly reminiscent of Freud, with, in addition, that crystalline clarity so characteristic of poets when they turn to prose. It is not only the style that evokes Freud, but by the case itself, with its interpretations, dreams, and the countless governesses, nannies, and maids who take turns in the lustful initiation of little Giannis T., it could well stand as the sixth clinical case from Freud's *Five Case Studies*, alongside "The Wolf Man," with which it shares the greatest affinity.[6]

As this first impression solidifies, its cracks begin to emerge. The differences from Freud's clinical monographs are numerous and structural, they go beyond the obvious. At a deeper level, however, one encounters deposits—constants—that pertain to fundamental choices. Both in Freud and in Embiricos, we observe how the questioning gaze upon reality, as it is deployed onto the multilayered discourse of the analysand—who in turn constructs a multilayered temporality—reveals their shared concern for a new, unprecedented passage through it, ever more productive, without end. The problem of the "primal scene" (*scène primitive*)—at the crossroads of fantasy and external and psychic reality—poses this question with a unique insistence, though in a way that is different for each of the two authors. Hence its frenzied pursuit.

Thus, although, as we have said, Embiricos' style in this text is anything but Surrealist, a second reading reveals the author's unwavering adherence to the Surrealist credo. Even in this text, he struggles—using different terminology—to render the truest version of reality: although here it is formally called "psychic" reality, his poems have no other motive than to make even the humblest fragment of reality worthy of such a title. A final reminder, once again, that Surrealism is not *une affaire de style* but *une affaire de vie*.

Reality. The primary tool and, at the same time, the ultimate goal of the Surrealists. But which reality? Not a coherent synthesis of nature, but a reality grafted on to the human gaze; a reality that, as it contains *contradiction*, is not "natural" in that sense, but rather one filled with passion, indeterminacy, and surprises.[7] If the Surrealists tasked themselves with engaging the most authentic mechanisms of the mind, it is because they had identified and articulated the functional relationship between what is called the material world and humankind. They had well understood that our undeniable sense of familiarity with the objects around us—whether animate or inanimate—the warmth and roundness of their forms, is due to the fact that they have taken on something from humankind, something from that primordial encounter with them, and this encounter is then continually repeated, deepening the familiarity. For this encounter, before any homeostasis that may emerge, imparts to them that touch that is both recognizable and familiar to humankind and which borders on the conceptual abstraction of materiality without contradicting it.

This is a first and perhaps less obvious point of contact between Surrealism and psychoanalysis, yet a fundamental one. It is to the latter that we owe the most reliable insights we have into what we might call the humanization of reality. As psychoanalysis dismantled the category of "object" in order to create a new one for its own purposes, it discovered therein traces of the human gaze. And within the human being, entire fragments of the world. Psychoanalysis recognized, in that primordial encounter we mentioned earlier, a genuinely electric contact, one that lays the groundwork for all subsequent ego identifications.

Surrealism heard this message, placing unwavering trust in the material world. It opened its eyes and ears to what dared not emerge into the light, for it recognized therein the most intriguing transformations of truth. It fearlessly approached the material world, seeing in it a sure guide for thought in its wanderings. Finally, even when it gazed into unexplored regions of life and mind, it remained anchored in the real, that is to say, in an entirely positive relationship with it, one that excluded all negation and nihilism.

In the field of art, such a perception of and approach to reality had striking consequences. A brilliant example, in our view, is a poem by Embiricos in *Oktana*, which unfolds as a symphony of human sensuality. Its theme is visual: a description of a maiden letting down her hair atop a rock. Yet, by the time the poem concludes, it has left tactile, gustatory, and other sensory impressions on the reader. But what ultimately surpasses the visual imagery is a subterranean auditory pandemonium fueled by the poet's extensive use of resonant alliterations and assonances. This, in retrospect, justifies its unexpected title, "*Korymvos*."[8]

The poem masterfully depicts an erotic object, speaking the language in which sensory stimuli find material expression. We have moved from the description of reality to the reality of the message.

Something else. The privileging of marginalized mental productions (such as absurdity, delirium, inconsistency, dreams, hallucinations) that is often attributed to Surrealism is to be relativized. This only seems to be the case when compared to their exclusion by the rationalist and positivist imperatives that have governed Western culture since the seventeenth century. Of greater importance was Surrealism's attempt to integrate the mind's authentic processes into artistic expression, and this endeavor can only be safeguarded by a force that keeps the logical, aesthetic, and moral filters at bay. With regard to the Surrealists' imitation of the unconscious, we might say that automatic writing, in its similarity to the analytic discourse that approximately obeys the fundamental rule, pursued two objectives: first, the highest possible degree of freedom, in the mathematical sense of the term;[9] and second, the immediate and instinctive transformation of psychic representations into to their verbal equivalents without the slightest delay, since it is precisely within such delay that censorship, in all of its forms, manages to enter through the backdoor. Yet Embiricos goes even further, which is without doubt one of the sharpest edges of his penetrating discourse: he spreads his writing like an inkblot, with loose semantics and a predominantly disjointed, paratactic syntax. The reader is invited to board a train full of promises, without knowing its destination—nor even being able to guess it. The title is enigmatic, and so the passenger does not even know at which station he has boarded. And yet there exists—like an entelechy—an inner coherence, in the same sense that the "primary process" (*processus primaire*), despite its anarchic succession of "presentations" (*représentations*), moves towards a point that attracts it like a magnet, what Freud calls the "purposive idea" (*représentation-but*). In fact, the more it resists the conscious pre-determination of its "purpose," the more inexorably it proceeds on a trajectory towards it. Embiricos' writing is structured around purposive words—some chosen for their associative potential, others for their sharp precision, and still some simply for their graceful sonority. The effect, in any case, is distinct: when at the turn of a phrase, we stumble upon such a *resonant word*, the text acquires the discontinuous rhythm of an eye that repeatedly catches on them. The poet entrusts to this rosary of words all the magical charge of his drives and fantasies, so that, as the beads multiply along the way, the endings of his poems often resemble a kind of erotic recomposition.

In the Text

"*Un cas de névrose obsessionnelle avec éjaculations précoces*" is built around the patient's life events and memories, as well as the associations and interpretations stemming from his three dreams. The narrative is largely guided by the analysand; that is, Embiricos allows its flow to follow his patient's associations rather than his own interventions, reserving for himself a more fluid position in terms of his roles. In a manner analogous to the structure of a literary work, he alternates between or simultaneously assumes the roles of narrator, reader, protagonist, or minor character. And there are times when he withdraws completely from the foreground, confining himself solely to the role of author. A dominant role, nonetheless, as he undertakes the task of organizing the narrative around the two vertical axes: the chronological (historical) and the "topographical" (conscious-unconscious) stratification. The dramatic elements, the use of historical tenses, but above all, the search for the primal scene—its progressive revelation, the unbroken suspense—gives the text an undeniably novelistic form. A novel does indeed exist here, but it is not the life of Giannis T. that is being narrated; rather, it is the protagonist's own investigation of the truth of this life. Novelistic time is inverted: we move backwards. The conclusion of the narrative coincides not with the happy or unhappy resolution of the hero's adventures, but with the final coming-into-focus of a hitherto blurry picture of reality—his own reality. This coming-into-focus will take place when the reconstruction of his personal mythology has been completed. Thus, to each moment of fictional time corresponds a horizontal cross-section of the whole story. Here, instead of a puzzle being progressively completed by an accumulation of elements and events, the puzzle is laid out before us from the outset and is continuously assembled and reassembled with a different configuration each time. The whole structure is reminiscent of those novels in which successive versions of the same events are presented in sequence.

The emphasis on memories and dreams—at the expense of fantasies, daydreams, slips, or hypotheses formulated by the patient—and the almost exclusively sexual nature of the material firmly situate this monograph within the most orthodox Freudian tradition. It is situated at quite a remove from similar works in the psychoanalytic literature (both contemporaneous and more recent), which have accustomed us to abundant explanations to the reader rather than interpretations to the analysand. Here, the analyst-narrator's communication with his audience is entrusted to Embiricos the writer, thanks, of course, to the practiced hand of the latter. That is to say, the very writing itself, in an indirect yet captivating way, often signals the progression of the treatment—sometimes even the countertransference dynamic—alongside the sporadic information given by Embiricos the psychoanalyst.

Let us examine this more concretely. It is not due to carelessness that, in the first, somewhat introductory section, nearly all verb tenses are used (historical present, imperfect, simple past, present perfect, pluperfect). These tenses, with their continuous shifting between each other, do not correspond to distinct temporal layers but rather overlap in terms of their placement within the narrative—only to eventually stabilize into a more rigorous use of past tenses. This initial section includes the presentation of the patient's request for treatment, a brief overview of the patient's history, and an incomplete list of symptoms—material that we have every reason to believe, even if this is not explicitly stated, corresponds roughly to the content of the preliminary interviews, when the analyst (here, Embiricos) has not yet, at least in theory, decided whether to accept the request, and has not yet "entered" into an analytic relationship. On the other hand, the complete lack of *je* (the first-person singular) in this part, which effectively causes the analyst to disappear behind the narrator, hints at Embiricos' deliberate choice to present the request along with the initial symptoms exactly as they were presented to him during the initial meetings, a mere transcription of them *without his personal intervention.* We can picture him in these preliminary meetings, seated motionless and expressionless in his chair, but above all silent, listening to the patient's words.

The metaphorical structuring of the text—because that is precisely what it is—becomes even more intriguing in the next section. The account of young

Giannis' erotic awakenings, which constitutes the content of this section, adopts the most banal, or rather, neutral, narrative form: a strict alignment of verb tenses (primarily the simple past, with the imperfect used where necessary), dialogue rendered in indirect speech, and a minimal use of "*shifters*" limited to the absolute minimum necessary. One might say that this is executed in the purest manner, untouched by the presence of the narrator, who is almost entirely absent. And as there is no discernible gap or variation in style this narrative unsettles the reader—who cannot forget that its narrator can ultimately only be the analysand—because it bears little resemblance to the type of speech typically uttered on the psychoanalytic couch.

Finally, if the presence of the narrator can only be guessed at, that of the analyst is *a fortiori* non-existent. There is no commentary that would betray the "second-degree" type of listening by the one to whom Giannis is addressing himself. Absent is any type of skepticism or disbelief. This is a different approach from Freud's, who isolates each narrated episode, each fantasy, each screen memory, commenting on them and often laying them on the Procrustean bed of theory (despite his claims to the contrary). Consequently, his narrative is more syncopated and labyrinthine, the presence of the analyst-interpreter-commentator never absent.

Let us not forget, however, that in writing his clinical cases Freud is constructing his theory. This forces him into a series of tricks and subtle maneuvers—as François Roustang has shown, by uncovering their covert, quasi-illicit operation[10]—in order to secure the reader's agreement.

Embiricos is working off of an already-established theoretical framework, which allows him to compose a better-oiled and less hesitant narrative. Yet this narrative, with all of its contradictory facets, still manages to express the reality of the therapeutic process. In the section we are considering, the clarity of the patient's memory can only be artificial. After all, we are not told how it entered the analytic space: are these screen memories, conscious or preconscious recollections? What is the extent of the analyst's constructions? These are nuances to which Freud, in "The Wolf-Man," attributes great significance. The uniform, neutral style obviously serves a purpose: to provide a counterpoint that accentuates what follows later, namely, the three dreams and the associations to them, which will ultimately lead to the emergence of the primal scene. Yet, this style serves a more "analytic," more unconscious function. In reality, the narrator has not disappeared (as is always the case); rather, he must be sought behind the absence of *je*, just as the analyst must be sought behind the absence of the psychoanalytic armchair; specifically, in this very distortion of the writing, which unsettles the reader, much like the presence of the human hand is inferred from the force exerted upon a natural form. This implicit presence is what makes the discourse interpretive, in a way that will become fully apparent in the next section. In general, a psychoanalytic text must intervene in its material with audacity—it must explain without dissipating contradiction, interpret where there are no obvious interpretations, describe with spontaneity, and even lapse into delirium with a touch of irony; it must set traps for the reader's imagination. The peculiarity of its subject matter compels it to adopt a distinctive rhetoric. Let's take another example from this paper: in the final pages, the constant shifts between direct and indirect speech make it impossible to discern where Giannis' words end and where the analyst's interpretations begin. But isn't this the deepest reality of the analytic relationship?

This narrative, which due to its linear condensation and temporal inelasticity could hardly be called novelistic—rather, it resembles the dry reading in court of the acts of indictment before the main trial begins—ends in a theatrical manner: "He [Giannis] swore upon the cross by kissing it, and the young maid entrusted him with her secret: 'It is your father . . .' she said, and left the room, hiding her face in her apron." Whereupon Embiricos makes his appearance on stage through a sudden shift in writing style. For the first time, the discourse is enlivened by the emotional reactions of the patient, as well as indications of his capacity for insight, or at least his attempts in that direction. The interpretative dimension suddenly becomes visible, and this is no accident. In fact, it is *necessary*, because the dropping of the curtain leads directly to the emergence of what is called the primal scene. The narrative task at this point can only be to highlight the rupture thus caused in Giannis' hitherto straightforward narrative. We thus observe an immediate dramatization. On one hand, brushstrokes are applied to color in the yet-pale figures in the drama: the love object is sullied (Maria—the maid—maintains a relationship with the father for money), and the father acquires traits (a womanizer) capable of provoking his son's jealousy and admiration alike. On the other hand, the son's description of the *coitus a tergo* he witnessed through the keyhole seems like something straight out of a horror film. Here is the harvest from a 12-line paragraph: *erotically pleasurable yet terrifyingly violent, slaughter, pain, torture, possessed by mania, enormous, monstrous and savagely lustful dog*. This writing is perfectly suited to the unique harshness that, according to Freud, all "trauma" has in its repetition. "This scene," said Giannis, "had unsettled him to an unimaginable degree. Yet, despite the anxiety and the deep sense of inferiority it instilled in him, its memory set him ablaze, he said, as though it were an extremely arousing thing, and it awoke within him the desire to see it again."

At the same time, the presence of Embiricos in his dual capacity intensifies; phrases such as "he says," "he tells me," "he added" crop up here and there, positioning both the subject of the utterance and the subject of the statements in their respective places. For the first time, the analysand is referred to as "my patient." The possessive pronoun could be seen as the cornerstone of the transference interpretation—one of the most classic of its kind—which is introduced on the very next page. At last, we see Embiricos in his most real form: a prop for the transference.

But, as if wanting to remind us of the distance necessary for such a narrative—a distance that his sudden entrance into the foreground might have misled us into thinking had not been maintained—he pauses and turns to theoretical sources (K. Abraham). Armed with the necessary arguments, he then proceeds with a reexamination of the same material, this time with a generous dose of interpretations, which, when communicated to the patient, cause a shift in course. Here, the writing style comes remarkably close to Freud's. This is not only found in the presence of certain phrases that one might swear one had encountered verbatim in Freud's work, such as: "I had the impression that behind the dramatic episode traumatic elements lay hidden beneath the more recent layers. These elements constituted, from within the deepest strata of his unconscious, the true source of his neurosis." If we attempt an analysis of the paragraph containing the interpretative hypothesis, we shall see how closely the arrangement of the meaning-bearing words resembles that which characterizes Freudian texts:

interpretation (*interprétation*)	(1)
fear (*peur*)	(2)
phrase (*phrase*)	(3)
active position (*orientation active*)	(4)
unconscious (*inconscientes*)	(5)
passive role (*rôle passif*)	(6)
passively (*passivement*)	(6)
penis (*verge*)	(7)
actively (*activement*)	(4)
phrase (*phrase*)	(3)
fear (*peur*)	(2)
penis (*verge*)	(7)
Interpretation (*interprétation*)	(1)
phrase (*phrase*)	(3)
passive (*passives*)	(6)
unconscious (*inconscientes*)	(5)

We observe the following: first these words—and they are quite numerous—are used at the beginning of the paragraph and repeated towards its end. Second, for some of them, the order of appearance is reversed. Third—though this is not evident here—words that were on the periphery of the previous paragraph now occupy the center of this one. These correspond respectively to what François Roustang has identified as Freud's dominant rhetorical devices, namely: *inclusion*, *chiasmus* or *hysteron-proteron*, and "*pericenter*," along with *concatenation* (the repetition at the beginning of a paragraph of the words at the end of the preceding one).[11]

The shift in the writing to such a multidimensional style, so radically different, seems, in retrospect, to cast an oblique light on the preceding narrative, without, however, depriving those earlier pages of their stylistic autonomy. Embiricos' second rewriting of the same theme serves as a reminder to the reader of the off-center balance inherent in analytic discourse. More than that, it validates what had already been subtly suggested by that seemingly unprepossessing account—namely the interpretative event between Embiricos and his patient. Indeed, this contrast is interpretative in the sense previously discussed, precisely because it reveals the actual function of the self-sufficiency that characterized Giannis' discourse at that stage of the analysis: it did not reveal, but concealed; it was not a speech-as-truth, but speech-as-screen that held truth prisoner. In the end, was his flawless coherence not one of those veils that, with its dense weave, Giannis, like a true obsessional, used to cover his objects?[12] We can now clearly see how interpretative analysis subverts discourse that is mobilized in the service of the resistances: the erotic involvement with Maria, a crucial pivot in Giannis' personal mythology, becomes for him a palimpsest of the primal scene. The void of the "unknown (male) other"[13] is filled with the only figure who could fill it: "It's your father . . ." A key phrase that opens a gap in this seamless discourse, pointing towards a forgotten memory, of which the present is merely a repetition: ". . . perhaps reality only takes shape within memory", as Proust says.

The emergence of the primal scene is now fully ripe not only psychoanalytically but also for the reader. A series of transformations in the writing are seen into motion to adapt it to what it has to say. If, up until this point, the text had been addressing a *reader*, it now demands a *spectator*. It is not surprising, then, that the author employs theatrical devices—one might even dare to say *stagecraft*—to draw the gaze toward the threshold between fantasy and memory, whence it will be afforded a glimpse of the "other" reality. Dreams with a phantasmagorical, even cosmopolitan, atmosphere take center stage one after another. The increasingly frequent use of the present tense immobilizes time, nailing it in place. Direct speech, at first timid but gradually asserting itself, takes over the recounting of the patient's words. A sleight-of-hand redistribution of roles and positions occurs: the description of the scene in which Giannis watches the governess masturbate has a lyrical quality that is unsettling, within a text that, while elegant, remains austere. Its vividness might lead one to suspect Embiricos' own taking part—not only in the voyeuristic pleasure of witnessing the sexually aroused young woman, but perhaps even in the act of peeping itself.[14]

Finally, for the first time, the narrator addresses the reader: "You might imagine the interpretative use I made of everything that . . ." And on the next page, "my patient" has become "our patient." Is this an implicit invitation to take part *from within* in the upcoming finale? An unconscious need for our "complicity" in the handling of this increasingly burdensome relationship? One thing is certain: the way the patient is named is never chosen at random. It appears to track both the fluctuations of the countertransference, and the shifting roles assumed alternately by the characters in the narrative, always in conjunction with the economy of the text. To take another example, the transition from the more frequent Giannis T. to the rarer Giannis, without the surname, does not suggest greater familiarity on the part of the narrator, as one might assume. This is proven by its almost-exclusive use in sections where Embiricos remains as uninvolved as possible, namely sections of the patient's memories, where it designates the protagonist of erotic adventures, the hero of his personal mythology, so to speak. On the contrary, it is the *reader* who experiences familiarity—or rather, sympathy—when reading about the "misfortunes of Giannis." This is a remarkably meticulous strategy on the author's part, and it extends beyond this useful emotional device. By restricting the use of "Giannis" to the aforementioned passages—where what the name refers to is less the subject of discourse and more the object in the hands of fate (read: *repetition*)—the author avoids employing the same term when Giannis is the *subject* of the enunciation (i.e., in its most demystifying function).

The Real Offspring of Imagination

Someone once likened poetic speech to *Grundsprache*, the "basic language" of President Schreber. It was spoken by the "birds" who were "souls," which in turn were "rays" that sent him the encrypted messages of divine will. In essence, it was a coded discourse built upon Schreber's deeply disturbed relationship with language, and, in turn, his language's relationship to external reality, a dialogue that has taught us more about human thought than numerous scholarly treatises ever could. This is something that often occurs when psychotic insight is paired, as in Schreber, with an uncommonly penetrating mind. The price, of course, is heavy: a splitting of the ego and its displacement into a realm of exile from which the basic language will be heard.

Not as a price to be paid, but rather as a kind of adolescent wanderlust, exile also exists in poetry—at least, this is the claim of someone who has dwelt in poetry for a long time, so we can only give credence to his words:

> The poem is exile, and the poet who belongs to it, belongs to the insatiable yearning of exile; he exists outside himself, far from his birthplace . . . this exile—the poem—makes him the wanderer, the one ever astray, the one deprived of stable presence and true dwelling.[15]

However, from the poet's exile, his words bring us "a life-giving breath of the sea" full of the musical pleasure of language and the wonder of images, allowing us to communicate—by killing off what the quotidian corrupts—with something more enduring. As in Schreber's world, where "divine miracles ('rays') always restored what had been destroyed, and therefore, as long as he remained a man, he is altogether immortal,"[16] so too does poetry restore shattered proportions and hurls memory through time, for the very reason that it is a fusion of the poet's personal mythology with the collective mythological tradition (what Freud calls "distorted vestiges of the wishful phantasies of whole nations, the *secular dreams* of youthful humanity"[17]). It is this, ultimately, that makes the poet's private dialogue with himself communicable to the reader.

The extent to which these two sources mutually nourish one another in Embiricos' work is evidenced not only in his personal reinterpretations of official myths (especially some of the last texts of *Amour Amour*, where the very themes themselves make evident the author's goal of reconnecting with humanity's self-awareness, as it was concisely articulated by some classical author). Rather, mythical elements abound throughout his poetic *oeuvre*; we see them coalesce each time into a narrative motif, taking shape as distinctly heterotopic inhabitants of thought—memories, echoes, sketches, fantasies, and so on. At the same time, through the mixing of verb tenses, the poem's present—the present moment in which the poet addresses the reader—projects the boundless, diachronic spectrum that the imagination was sweeping across at the very moment of the poem's conception.

This aspect of poetry holds particular interest (to which we will return shortly), because it helps clarify the deep resonance that the primal scene holds for a poet-psychoanalyst. It serves as the link that magically connects, for each individual, the "common phylogenetic heritage" with the "accidents" of their personal history. For, no matter how we approach it, Embiricos' insistence on the primal scene in Giannis' analysis is striking and cannot be attributed (or at least not solely) to his dogmatic adherence to Freudian paradigms. There is also this: once it emerges, the case study concludes—it is followed neither by an interpretation nor a synthetic reconsideration based on this important new element, as one might naturally expect. This gives it an autonomous value, as if it had no other purpose than that of any other resolution: namely to meet the expectations of Embiricos as an analyst and our own as readers.[18]

What's going on here? We assume that Embiricos is particularly sensitive to the mythical dimension of the primal scene as a concept. Mythical, because it splits the individual's history in two: as the metonymy of the primordial communion with the object of desire (which is neither the breast, nor the vulva, nor the penis, but the forever-lost object), it acts as a catalyst in sexuality "to destroy the unyielding bondage of geometry with another geometry—this one without limits" (M. Leiris). It organizes psychic space into a new arrangement around the void, the *ellipse*, which will forever symbolize that lost object and attract an infinite number of others—though none will be anything more than futile substitutes for the original. Here, too, the role of fantasy is decisive: it is fantasy that fragments any auditory or visual image the child receives—a sudden awakening in the night, or even a half-open door. Fantasy fragments it, detaches it from the context of the given situation and—like the photographic shutter in the eponymous poem from *Oktana*—"*transforms a static moment (let's say, a fixed one) into an undulating dance of hours and supple bodies in rhythmic harmony, into a tangible and quivering embodiment of every vision, of every desire*."

Freud describes this mechanism in a clear and straightforward formulation in "The Wolf Man," where he extensively explores the primal scene:

> Wherever experiences fail to fit in with the hereditary [*i.e., phylogenetic*] schema, they become remodeled in the imagination—a process which might very profitably be followed out in detail. It is precisely such cases that are calculated to convince us of the independent existence of the schema.[19]

We might see the primal scene as a unique fold in reality, meaning that incontestable material facts are displaced along the axis that connects the individual to humanity's past as a species. The key to this displacement lies in the final sentence, which asserts that the phylogenetic scheme exists independently of individual variations in events—yet, it does not, on its own, have exclusive authority over their consequences. In short, the facts may be what they are, but there also exist the psychic residue of millennia of cultural life—something no less real, and indeed, no less material.

The primal scene thus becomes a model for the metaphorical relationship between the reality of events and the other reality—psychic reality. And perhaps it is at this point that we should seek the explanation for the fascination it holds for Embiricos, who, as a Surrealist, rejects the traditional opposition between the two realities. Indeed, as far as poetic creation was concerned, Surrealism made no distinction between the two, believing that through their convergence, art could escape the ephemeral. An unconscious conduit is necessary to transfer material from the phylogenetic reservoir into the fleeting nature of a particular experience or individual inspiration.

Of course, between the theoretical position and its practical realization lies a difficulty, one that is inherent in writing itself due to its artificial nature. Writing is a luxury activity, something that is added as a "surplus" to the other activities of life. However, for it to fulfill its mission—to speak about life in a way that nothing else can—it is not enough for it to find a justification. It must become an absolutely necessary activity, an utterly pressing need, like making love, having social interactions with others, or knowing what time it is. But this can only happen if the work consumes one's entire existence: if it steals the woman you love, if it makes socializing with one's friends impossible (let us recall Proust), and upends your very sense of time.

In any case, the point is that art—living, true art—exists in a continuous, entirely material exchange with the artist's life. This is the channel that grants it access to material reality. For let us not forget that art deals with material things, not mere symbols—something that applies, of course, to Embiricos' poetry as well. As he himself states when describing the trajectory he followed in pursuit of the greatest expressive effectiveness, the poem finds its eternal, timeless elements within matter itself and its transformations.[20] The play of words is a constant back-and-forth between objects—in their material substance and practical function—and their symbols.

Let us see how this is achieved in a specific example. "Land of Landscape" (in *Amour Amour*) handles its subject in a material way: it describes trees, rocks, and hills—it does not merely list symbols. And yet, we are constantly presented with the figure of a voluptuous woman beckoning us to touch her. The erotic effect is due much less to the two or three overtly sexual associations made by Embiricos, and far more to his use of imagery such as *a space opens up . . . in a series of harmonious folds, bare, covered, protuberance, deeply folded, smoothly curved swellings and alternating foamless hollows, tufts*[21]—all of which attribute the natural landscape the geometry of a naked body. The land described does not *resemble* a woman, it *is* a woman.

In a highly paradoxical way, his poetry—perhaps all poetry?—aims at the atemporal by working within the interval that separates two temporalities: the thing from the symbol. Here, one cannot avoid linking poetic language to desire, an association that makes the paradox less puzzling. If poetry possesses something of desire's incorruptibility, it is perhaps because both move in the same in-between space, where memory constructs analogies. This is where desire finds its objects: from the breast as a lactating organ, to the breast nestled inside the orifice of the child's mouth, completing its form. Or, if this example lacks eloquence, from the tangible materiality of an undergarment to the phallic symbol. This space is "tunneled" by fantasy.

The Surrealists, better than anyone else, convinced us of the following: that the world of fantasy is not external, or in addition to, the realm of things, and that, therefore, its most fruitful exploration requires not an additive but a subtractive act; by eliminating a thousand intermediary words, the metaphor is propelled forward. Is this not precisely what Embiricos does when he forces the most heteroclite words into an unnatural union?

When one writes, one tries to penetrate reality and describe its hidden regions. When one writes metaphorically—that is, when one's hand is guided by the laws of fantasy—one searches for objects with greater precision: one constructs objects of desire within reality. We know from the commonest experience—not only that of perversion—that for such an endeavor, no process is more effective than fantasy. This also makes it a crucial testimony to the intimacy between man and the real that surrounds him, as we described at the beginning. Isn't it fascinating—and, in a way, almost like a gesture of courtesy on reality's part—that fragments of it can become objects of human desire?

An anamnesis by Giannis T. vividly illustrates the plasticity of fantasy, how it exploits events, appropriates them, and ultimately reshapes them according to its own logic, distancing itself from their literal level. This is the scene with the little dog—an original piece in an erotic anthology. One day, upon entering his mother's boudoir, young Giannis found her lying there, reading. At his appearance, his mother made a sudden movement, and her little Pekingese dog sprang out from between her legs onto the floor, slightly lifting up the hem of the robe she was wearing. She seemed flustered, and addressing the little dog, said: "Bobby, aren't you ashamed of yourself, you tore my robe . . . You deserve a beating!"

Giannis never found out exactly what had happened between his mother and the Pekinese. He was left, as we were, with the scabrous doubt hanging in the air, as if to add even more eroticism to this scene which is already permeated with it. What was of importance to Giannis (and to the subject at hand) is his mother's guilty look, not whether it was justified—as demonstrated by the following: despite the ambiguity—or perhaps because of it—this incident, when recalled to memory, is what designates his mother as an erotic object, since it is his only memory that concerns her. One might even suppose that a less ambiguous spectacle, by imprisoning the imagination, would have produced a memory with a milder affective charge—much like how the most unbearable eroticism can be measured in the shared glances of two almost-lovers, while the sex act itself wipes it away.

Thus, this is how the object is constituted within the field of fantasy. The voluptuous element that captures Giannis' desire could be the fleeting, staccato gaze that momentarily leaves the book to inspect the disarray of her clothing, or perhaps a brief flush that may have unsettled her face—in short, anything that, however fleetingly, suggests the desire of the other. This alone is enough; the evidence of reality is unnecessary, since in any case only fantasy can offer the promise of pleasure.

From that point on,[22] Giannis' fantasy glides over uncertainty and expands outwards to embrace ever broader—yet monstrous—speculations:

> I don't know what happened in my mother's boudoir, and I repeat that most probably nothing happened, but for a long time, I could not free my mind of that suspicion, and then another suspicion was added to it, namely that perhaps my mother would allow the Pekingese to penetrate her, and also my father's big hunting dog of whom she was also very fond.

And a little further down:

> . . . [A]fter having discovered that his governess masturbated, he often wondered (with the same reactions of anxiety and guilt) whether his mother didn't also masturbate. And he said that he often wondered if his mother hadn't in fact died of pneumonia, but rather because of his father's brutal penetration, on one hand, but also because of her masturbation and what she was doing with the dogs, on the other.

We can see here, apart from the typically obsessional components (doubt, guilt, and above all the deathly outcome as the only conceivable resolution of desire), we also recognize the familiar fertility of fantasy. As it unfolds, this fantasy is reproduced in ever-new scenarios, offering the subject endless permutations to allow him access to those events, all the while leaving the ego blissfully undisturbed, since, of course, it wants nothing to do with any of this. Embiricos' interpretation, in which he points out to his patient the projective mechanisms at work, does no more than bring to light that which is unconsciously latent in his fantasy, namely, *the multiple ways in which he enters the fantasy as a subject of desire*:

> I also told Giannis T. that already at that point, as later, he wanted to take the place of the dog in what he suspected it did to his mother (cunnilingus, coitus), acts that he wanted to perform himself, but that whether or not his mother had allowed herself to be licked by the dogs, he could not accept as his own the desires that he projected onto her.

Without a doubt, the fact that fantasy can and does, in a way, dominate one's perception of the material world and interactions with it, stems from this maximum freedom the subject exercises over its disguises. There remains an open question as to whether this freedom is something that poetry exploits, and, if so, through what process. This is certainly a legitimate hypothesis if one considers that poetic language is cyclical—it has neither a center nor a fixed referent, nor does it communicate anything in the conventional sense. Where is the subject located in an Embiricos poem? Kafka once stated—with satisfaction, no less—that for him, literary production truly began once he was able to replace *Ich* (I) with *Er* (he—impersonal).

We are not talking about the usual and harmless phenomenon of daydreaming—imagining oneself in the place of another, doing something, where, under the cover of an intact sense of identity, I allow myself every conceivable substitution. Fantasy, on the contrary, is far from innocent. Thanks to its directorial abilities, it overdetermines the subject within a web of relations, but it also annihilates, or rather erases, the subjective point of view altogether. The prototypical fantasy we are given is "A Child Is Being Beaten," not "I Am Being Beaten." Perhaps that is why Freud places such deep stock in this fantasy. Beyond granting it a theoretical status, as he does with all of his concepts, here, he also elevates it to the status of theory itself. In one point in "Analysis Terminable and Interminable," he says that "if we are asked by which methods and means this result is achieved, it is not easy to find an answer. We can only say: '*So muss denn doch die Hexe dran!*'—the Witch Meta-psychology." He adds, "without metapsychological speculation and theorizing—*I had almost said 'phantasying'*—we shall not get another step forward."[23] Almost scandalous.

The meaning is clear: if you want to know the real, you must move along its borders. To do so, you must push your own limits as far as possible. Thus, you have every reason not to dismiss fantasy as an agent of deception. On the contrary, fantasy challenges the intrinsic limitations of knowledge, as it compensates for a reality that is absent from your personal history. And this, Embiricos was enough of a psychoanalyst to have known, and enough of a poet to have pursued.

Notes

1 First published in *Psychanalysē kai Ellada—Stoicheia, theseis, erōtēmata* [Psychoanalysis and Greece—Evidence, Positions, Questions], ed. Thanasēs Tzavaras (Athens: Etaireia Spoudōn Neoellēnikou Politismou kai Genikēs Paideias [Society for the Study of Modern Greek Culture and General Education], 1984), 107–30.
2 Sacha Nacht, "Le masochisme: Étude clinique et thérapeutique," *Revue Française de Psychanalyse* 14, no. 3 (1950): 331–66; also published in English translation as chapter 1 of the present volume.
3 More correctly, published. He also wrote the other texts contained in the present volume, which are now seeing the light of day.
4 As in this entire document, used in the broader sense of a literary exercise.
5 Pierre-Yves Bourdil, "Entre chien et chat: la parole par elle-même," *Poétique* no. 45 (1981): 82. The author, in turn, cites in a footnote the following passage from Martin Heidegger, "The different kinds of origin of S[ubject] and P[redicate] perhaps most sharply illuminate the inner questionability of the basic structure of logic, long unquestioned, the *logos* and the *proposition*," in *Schelling's Treatise on the Essence of Human Freedom*, trans. J. Stambaugh (Athens, OH: Ohio University Press, 1985), 78.
6 Struck by this resemblance, we decided to take a closer look at the text. And so, this became the occasion for a peculiar and "symptomatic" reading. The text at hand is the edited, written transference of that experience—and nothing else.
7 "At this point, let us consider what new elements Surrealism introduced: it expanded the concept of reality by incorporating contradiction, broadened the notion of structure by including the disorder of objective 'chance,' and finally, extended the boundaries of language to include its non-logical aspects." M. Chryssanthopoulos, "The Emergence of Greek Surrealism (Literary and Intellectual Origins)," Unpublished PhD dissertation, University of Birmingham, 33, 1979.
8 Translator's note: "*Korymvos*" can mean (a) the uppermost point (of a ship, a mountain, a hairknot atop the head); (b) the edge of a tomb; (c) a cluster of fruit, particularly ivy fruit. It also hints at sexual climax.
9 Freedom, whose role nevertheless remains obscure and whose authority is uncertain. For what determinism have they thus cast off their shackles? Who would claim that the "chance object" is truly random? If trusting chance means trusting the laws of chance, then one way to increase your freedom—and certainly not the most foolish one—is to learn their logic. We will cite an example from a movement on the opposite end of the spectrum from Surrealism: the OuLiPo (*Ouvroir de littérature potentielle* [Workshop of potential literature]) movement, which through the accumulation of (often complex) deliberate constraints on form, experimented on literary structures to create new ones, as well as new techniques in

poetry. The OuLiPians, among whom was Raymond Queneau—this as evidence of the seriousness of their intentions and the effectiveness of their prescriptions—did not feel that their creative freedom was restricted by the syntactic restraints they placed upon themselves. On the contrary, they significantly expanded the horizons of literature; specifically, they transformed constraints into a source of inspiration, thus promoting a modern, one might say "materialist," conception of literature. Although they followed an opposite path, their aim was similar to that of Surrealism. After all, many of them emerged out of Surrealist groups. But there were also many mathematicians among them, and this is no accident (such as Georges Perec; his masterpiece novel, *La Vie Mode d'Emploi*, a mature OuLiPian effort, is an example of imaginative construction and a product of the highest degree of freedom). It is speculated that mathematics is, as a mental process, very akin to literature. In any case, one thing is certain: it requires a robust imagination. The great mathematician Hilbert was asked how one of his colleagues had managed to become a writer. His response: "Oh, it's simple. He didn't have enough imagination for mathematics, but he had just enough for novels."

10 François Roustang, "Du chapitre VII," *Nouvelle Revue de Psychanalyse* no. 16 (Autumn 1977): 65–95. A remarkable analysis of Freudian style in general.

11 François Roustang, "Du chapitre VII," *Nouvelle Revue de Psychanalyse* no. 16 (Autumn 1977): 85. The author attempts to show that Freud's style, among other things, is organized in the image of the theoretical system it expresses, and that occurs to a greater degree than in other writers; his system, being itself discursive, imposes this upon him. With its predominant syntactic forms being *parataxis* (the syntax of the unconscious, but also of poetry) and secondarily *hypotaxis* (typical of interpretation), his text mirrors unconscious mechanisms and dream work. Of course, it is difficult to say to what extent all of this is a result of Freud's conscious choices. Roustang, however, argues that what is important is to view his phrasing as reflective of the assembly of the psychic apparatus itself. The overwhelming use of such syntactic techniques makes Freudian writing "that mixture of slowness and acceleration, continuity and interruption. The frequent repetition of the entire preceding process gives the impression of a return to the starting point, yet the sudden introduction of new elements creates the opposite impression—that the overall perspective has profoundly shifted. Thus, many paragraphs take the following form: they initially appear to unfold in a linear fashion, stumble on a difficulty, seize upon a hypothesis or a conjecture, and ultimately bend back to return to the starting point, yet now laden with the journey they have traversed. Linearity imposes circularity upon itself, for a return down the same path can only occur via detours."

12 "A veil, both transparent and impenetrable, seems to separate the obsessional from the object of his desire. However he names it—whether a blue wall, a wall of cotton or of stone—for him, as he himself declares, it is *a glass sphere* that isolates him from reality." (Serge Leclaire, "L'Obsessionnel et son désir," *Évolution psychiatrique* no. 3 (1959): 383).

13 "In the throes of disappointment, and feeling inferior to that unknown 'other,' he once again demanded that she tell him who that man was, but the young servant girl began to laugh, and as always, stubbornly refused to reveal the name to him."

14 Indeed, the description in question seems straight out of Embiricos' poem "*Polles phores tēn nychta*" [Oftentimes at night] in *Oktana*; this is what the use of two characteristically "Embirican" words suggested to us. This poem could well be seen as a drawn-out primal scene with multiple variations. We note that the few passages in the text that suddenly adopt this embellished style all pertain to sexual activities by third parties as they being observed by Giannis (i.e., they are copies of the primal scene). Besides the one just mentioned, the others include the brutal description of the "unnatural" sex act between the father and the maid, the scene with the mother and the little dog, and the embrace of the wet-nurse and her "lover."

15 Maurice Blanchot, *L'Espace littéraire* (Paris: Gallimard, 1955), 322.

16 From the expert report compiled in 1899 by Dr. Weber. See "Psycho-Analytic Notes on an Autobiographical Account of a Case of Paranoia," in *Standard Edition of the Complete Psychological Works of Sigmund Freud* (hereafter *S.E.*), vol. 12 (London: Hogarth), 17.

17 Translator's note: "Creative Writers and Day Dreaming," *S.E.*, vol. 9, 152.

18 The second is sustained by the first, which loses none of its intensity until it comes to fruition: ". . . I had the impression that the primal scene was still escaping us"; "I momentarily believed that we were possibly going to see the memory of the primal scene . . . rise up from infantile amnesia." And again, "I had the impression that the primal scene was still escaping us."

19 Sigmund Freud, "From the History of an Infantile Neurosis," *S.E.*, vol. 17, 119. London, UK: The Hogarth Press.

20 "[I]f I could use, in the spheres of poetic creation, the same process that makes the flowing of the falling water such a rich, fascinating and indisputable reality, instead of describing this flowing." In Andreas Embiricos "Amour Amour," in *Amour Amour*, trans. Nikos Stangos and Alan Ross (Copenhagen and Los Angeles: Green Integer, 2003), 17.

21 Andreas Embiricos, "Amour Amour," in *Amour Amour*, trans. Nikos Stangos and Alan Ross (Copenhagen and Los Angeles: Green Integer, 2003), 52.

22 "At the moment of climax [*jouissance*], [pleasure] would simply be out of the picture if fantasy did not intervene to sustain it with the very discord to which it succumbs. Stated differently, fantasy provides the pleasure that is characteristic of desire." Jacques Lacan, "Kant with Sade," in *Ecrits*, trans. Bruce Fink (New York: W. W. Norton, 2006), 652.

23 Sigmund Freud, "Sigmund Freud," *S.E.*, vol. 23, 225 (italics ours). London, UK: The Hogarth Press.

Chapter 10

". . . Like All Women Like Herself, Like Alcmene . . ."

Female and Male Homosexuality in the Work of Embiricos

Nikos Sigalas

This article examines the way in which homosexuality is integrated into the erotic writings of Embiricos. I am not claiming that homosexuality occupies a central place in his work; rather, I believe it occupies a place of central importance in his work because of the prohibitions, stigma, and social condemnation of which it was the object. The way homosexual relationships are incorporated into the broader spectrum of relationships that constitute Embiricos' erotic writings is thus indicative of the latter's moral and theoretical underpinnings. I consider that what Embiricos wrote about homosexuality provides a direct key to unlocking his erotic literary production.

Before turning to the main subject of this article, I will touch on two points that may help in understanding it more fully. The first concerns the relationship between Embiricos' erotic writings and the "law." The second concerns the relationship between psychoanalysis and homosexuality.

"Laws Do Not Always Repress"

Embiricos first conceived the idea of writing an erotic text, or more precisely, of describing various erotic encounters, in his piece "Hoi horizontes ē hē phainomenologia tou erōtos" ("The Horizons or the Phenomenology of Eros").[1] Here, he depicts a series of erotic scenes that a passerby, endowed with acute perception and imaginative powers, perceives taking place around him as he follows a long road. The scenes encompass different facets of the phenomenon of Eros, enacted in secrecy and at times unlawfully, since "marble barriers and cement barriers rise up here and there." These barriers represent the prohibitions, the laws that set limits and constrain the freedom of Eros. Yet, as the passerby-psychoanalyst-surrealist poet observes (who, like another Hegel, is able to deduce from phenomena the universal becoming that occurs with and beyond them), "the laws do not always repress."[2]

The aphorism "the laws do not always repress" recurs periodically, like a refrain, throughout the text, underscoring its theoretical foundations. The "phenomenology of Eros" aspires both to describe the present reality of Eros and to envision its future development, in the manner that Hegel envisions the becoming of Spirit in his *Phenomenology*. These two dimensions, the descriptive and the visual, coexist, though they remain distinct, within Embiricos' erotic project. On the one hand, Embiricos describes what *exists*. On the other, he envisions the coming liberation of Eros. The reader must be careful not to assume that both dimensions represent his personal propositions. The phenomenon of Eros is described as it is, in all its forms—including some that Embiricos himself does not endorse, such as extreme sadism.[3] The vision, when articulated clearly, represents his own proposal. This distinction is one of the principal keys to understanding Embiricos' erotic writings, which presuppose a dynamic conception of time and a horizon of expectation.

Embiricos' "phenomenology of Eros" serves as the theoretical canvas of his erotic writings. This "phenomenology" is, pragmatically, from the first text in which it is introduced, a meditation on the law: "The laws do not always repress." As we shall see, a reflection on the law underlies Embiricos' entire erotic literary oeuvre. On this point, Embiricos joins some of the most important writers and thinkers of the interwar period, particularly in Germany and Austria, where psychoanalysis itself was born, namely Franz Kafka, Thomas Mann, Stefan Zweig, Joseph Roth, and Walter Benjamin, who, among many others, continually pondered the relation of the human being to the law, both from a social and metaphysical perspective.

The law and legal categories, moreover, lie at the foundation of Max Weber's sociology, while jurists and constitutional theorists such as Carl Schmidt, Hans Kelsen, and Franz Neumann were, at that time, central points of reference throughout the German-speaking intellectual world. So much so, in fact, that Freud invited Kelsen to publish a commentary on his *Group Psychology and the Analysis of the Ego* in *Imago*. Out of their exchange emerged the concept of the superego, which owes much to legal theory and, indeed, is essentially borrowed from it. For Kelsen, "the legal order is an order of coercion" (*Die Rechtsordnung ist eine Zwangsordnung*). The Freudian superego, in turn, is the internalization of coercion and, by extension, of guilt—the mechanism through which laws become internalized. Freud, however, took a decisive step beyond Kelsen and the logic of "pure" law that he espoused: he held that guilt is not merely the result of transgression but may itself generate transgression. Guilt (and thus the superego, in this context) is therefore not only a consequence or limit of criminality; it can also serve as its motive, producing criminality, as in the case of sadism. This constitutes Freud's invaluable critique of pure law, which lies in the background of his theory of the superego.[4]

The "barriers" and "laws" of which Embiricos speaks thus have a dual dimension. On the one hand, they refer to the actual laws that societies and governments impose in order to set limits on human erotic behavior; on the other, they refer to the internalized laws (the prohibitions, the taboos) that the individual imposes upon himself, that the superego imposes upon the id.

Psychoanalysis and Homosexuality

Let us now briefly examine how psychoanalysis has approached homosexuality. This is a complex subject with an extensive bibliography. A landmark text is Freud's 1920 essay "The Psychogenesis of a Case of Homosexuality in a Woman."[5] In this work, Freud refuses to categorize homosexuality as a degeneration or an abnormality along with the sexologists of his time. For Freud, homosexuality is not an "unnatural" sexual orientation, since, for him, all human beings are bisexual; their bisexuality simply remains latent in most cases. By restricting their erotic choices exclusively to individuals of the opposite sex, heterosexual people are repressing their bisexual nature. In a sense, exclusively homosexual individuals do the same, limiting their choice of erotic object to members of the same sex. In either case, according to Freud, these are Oedipal productions of the erotic self.[6]

In psychoanalytic terms, in the case of female homosexuality, we are dealing with an early fixation (*Fixierung*) on the mother, resulting from a disappointment with the father. In male homosexuality, by contrast, we are dealing with an "negative Oedipus complex": an identification with the mother arising from an inability to possess her—an inability to compete with the father and other men, and an acceptance of the passive role and passive pleasure.

Freud therefore does not consider homosexuality or, indeed, any of the other resolutions of the Oedipus complex to be psychic structures that can be transformed through treatment. The resolutions of the Oedipus complex constitute the unalterable givens of an analytic treatment. Psychoanalysts, therefore, should not attempt to "correct" homosexuality, as psychiatrists of the time generally sought to do.

From an ontogenic perspective, Freud holds that the homosexual individual has his own fate within civilization—a tragic fate, owing to the exclusion to which he is subjected. Yet, this destiny can be compensated through creativity and sublimation, to which homosexuals often resort, given the difficulties they face in realizing and gaining acceptance for their erotic choices. The homosexual individual thus becomes a creator. For Freud, he is *the* creator *par excellence*, the quintessential bearer of culture within society, as evidenced in his 1910 study of Leonardo da Vinci.[7] Freud elaborated these ideas more explicitly in 1935, in a well-known letter to an American woman whose son was homosexual:

> Homosexuality is assuredly no advantage, but it is nothing to be ashamed of, no vice, no degradation, it cannot be classified as an illness; we consider it to be a variation of the sexual function produced by a certain arrest of sexual development. Many highly respectable individuals of ancient

> and modern times have been homosexuals, several of the greatest men among them (Plato, Michelangelo, Leonardo da Vinci, etc.). It is a great injustice to persecute homosexuality as a crime and cruelty too. If you do not believe me, read the books of Havelock Ellis.[8]

In order to grasp how radical Freud's views on homosexuality were at the time, one need only consider the reactions they provoked among psychoanalysts, particularly in the English-speaking world. A turning point came in 1921, when a dispute erupted within the committee that secretly governed the International Psychoanalytic Association, over whether homosexuals should be permitted to become psychoanalysts. The Viennese group around Freud, represented chiefly by Otto Rank, maintained that there was no reason to exclude homosexuals, "just as we cannot accept the fact that homosexuals are persecuted by the law." By contrast, the Berlin group led by Karl Abraham was in favor of their exclusion, arguing that homosexuals could not be admitted to their ranks since psychoanalysis was incapable of "curing" them. The issue was ultimately decided by the position taken by the head of the British society, Ernest Jones, who was also president of the International Psychoanalytic Association (IPA). Jones declared that homosexuality is "a repugnant crime: if one of our members committed it, we would be seriously discredited."[9]

As a result, homosexual individuals were excluded from the IPA for many decades. The situation regarding homosexuality in fact worsened after Freud's death, under the influence of his daughter Anna, who adopted an explicitly homophobic stance and—unlike her father—maintained that homosexuals should be considered ill and subjected to treatment. This became, moreover, the dominant trend within the North American psychoanalytic societies after the war, whose influence within the IPA grew significantly. Even in France, after the war, homosexuals were barred from training analyses, and analysts sought to "help" them become heterosexual. The sole exception, on both counts, was Jacques Lacan and the *École Freudienne de Paris* (EFP), which he founded in 1964.

"A Case of Unconscious Homosexuality"

We must take these facts into account in order to understand how Embiricos approached the question of homosexuality in his erotic writings, which he composed while still practicing as a psychoanalyst. An additional important element is a study Embiricos began writing in French but left unfinished—most likely because it coincided with the period when he was forced to close his analytic practice—entitled "A Case of Unconscious Homosexuality."[10] This is the case study of a treatment he conducted with analysand Petros L., who initially consulted him for sexual impotence. Since the text remains incomplete, we cannot fully grasp the direction of the treatment, which, at least at an initial level, aimed at helping the analysand become conscious of his homosexuality ("*philhomophylia*").[11]

Embiricos' text is particularly interesting from a theoretical standpoint, since his interpretation of Petros L.'s homosexuality does not strictly follow the conventional Freudian path of the "negative Oedipus complex." Instead, it focuses on the fixation with the mother that occurs during the oral stage. This point is significant because in *Group Psychology and the Analysis of the Ego*, Freud notes that "at the very beginning, in the individual's primitive oral phase, object-cathexis and identification are no doubt indistinguishable from one another."[12] In other words, in the very text where Freud introduces the theory of identification, he points to the possibility of a form of identification that does not constitute an obstacle to desire, as other forms do, but rather coexists with it.[13]

"The patient is profoundly fixated upon his mother, and his libido seeks satisfactions in a pregenital manner, along oral and anal lines," writes Embiricos.[14] This sentence gives us a key for stepping beyond the conventional, surface level of the text (whose intended readership was the conservative milieu of the Paris Psychoanalytic Society [SPP] of the time) in order to reach Embiricos' own psychoanalytic theory. Within this ambiguous web between desire *for* the mother and identification *with* her, the psyche of Petros L. is trapped: through his masturbatory practices, "Petros L. . . . seeks not only to passively take pleasure from his mother, but also, by feeling and experiencing all of her sensations, to take pleasure from his father's penis as she does."[15] It is, then, a "conflictual" homosexuality, as Embiricos calls it, one that makes him simultaneously his wife's dependent and oppressor.

In this text, Embiricos speaks of an "inversion" of Petros' Oedipal complex, which, nonetheless, does not occur according to Freud's description of it: that is, anaclitically, as a result of the subject's failure to possess the mother. Instead, Embiricos emphasizes the importance of a "primary identification" with the mother. To this, he adds the Oedipal rivalry with the father, which Petros is unable to tolerate. In sum: the attentive reader can discern the outlines of an original and distinctive psychoanalytic theory for its time, one that Embiricos sought to conceal, given the exigencies of the prevailing circumstances (namely, the recognition of the Greek Psychoanalytic Society), behind a mask of strict Freudian orthodoxy.

I now turn to Embiricos' earliest text in which homosexual love is depicted: the story of the schoolteacher Maria, which forms the second part of the multifaceted piece "Anatolē" ("East"), and which later reappears in expanded form in *Ho Megas Anatolikos* (*The Great Eastern*).[16] The story of the schoolteacher Maria may, in fact, be regarded as the matrix of *The Great Eastern*, as it is the first and only episode of the novel to have been written prior to the novel itself. The title "Anatolē" itself foreshadows that of *The Great Eastern*.

". . . Like All Women Like Herself, Like Alcmene . . ."

The story unfolds roughly as follows: Maria, a private tutor from Athens, represses her homosexual libido, which at this particular moment in her life is expressed through her love for her young pupil, Irene, the greatest of all the loves she has ever felt—though never consummated. In reverie, at dawn, whilst still in bed, Maria reflects upon her love for Irene and the "Cyclopean barriers" that have prevented her, with one sole exception, from expressing her love for other girls. Within Maria's reverie, her life story gradually unfolds.

In summary: Maria had a bad relationship with her parents, especially with her father, who inspired in her both fear and revulsion (a basic Freudian motif in the Oedipal structure of female homosexuality). Maria's life knows a brief moment of happiness when her older cousin Alcmene comes to live with her and introduces her to love. But Alcmene's suicide, following the discovery of their relationship and the brutal beating inflicted upon her by Maria's father, brings Maria's erotic life to an abrupt end. From that moment on, she is never again able to show her feelings to any girl. "A part of herself," rigid and unyielding, becomes "a barrier" against the wave that the rest of her being represents. This "rigid" part, "the barriers that rise up," are the internalized laws, the superego. Her only exception and consolation is frequent masturbation and the recollection of that earlier time (before Alcmene's suicide) "when no barrier held her back." Having lived twenty years "without consummating a love," Maria longs for Alcmene and wishes "that she could do with Irene what Alcmene once did with her," wishes "that she could be like all women like herself, who—regardless of what is permitted or forbidden—manage sooner or later to find satisfaction, whatever the world may say, whatever the rules may say, whatever the laws may say!"[17] "The laws do not always repress," as we are reminded of the refrain from *Horizons*.

This passage clearly points towards the moral horizon of the text, the horizon of the psychoanalytic cure, of which the text is, in a sense, an extension (and from which it may indeed draw). The schoolteacher Maria is called upon to overcome both the internal and external "barriers," to act as Alcmene did, "like all women like herself . . . whatever the world may say, whatever the rules may say, whatever the laws may say!"

With this exhortation, Embiricos expresses the most progressive positions of psychoanalysis concerning homosexuality, like Otto Rank, when he held that psychoanalysts "cannot accept that homosexuals are persecuted by the law." As I have already noted, the story of the schoolteacher Maria essentially constitutes the point of departure for *The Great Eastern*, in whose first chapter Maria and Irene reappear. In the version found in *The Great Eastern*, the reflections of the schoolteacher Maria take on an even more pronouncedly declarative tone. Maria reflects:

> This good and honorable teacher, Maria, simply belonged to an erotic minority within the vast erotic majority that surrounded her; yet, her peculiarity was no less erotic. Her homosexuality, therefore, having its own justification, could very well coexist with the heterophilia of orthodox lovers, since it was not immoral before God, but only in the opinion of the

> moralists—for God, *in His knowledge*, had allowed her to be "thus," since her disposition was *thus* by nature. Thus, insofar as she did not set herself against the majority, she too could fulfill, *realize*, make her homosexuality an *accomplished fact* through her actions with Irene, or with any other young woman or girl—just like all women like herself, somewhere, in a small corner of Pan's boundless embrace, without troubling the loves and feelings of his orthodox children.[18]

What struck me most in the two excerpts above, from "Anatolē" and *The Great Eastern*, was the phrase "like all women like herself." It brought to mind Cavafy's note:

> The wretched laws of society—deriving neither from hygiene nor from judgement—diminished my work. They bound my expression; they prevented me from giving light and emotion to those who are made like me.

This note from Cafafy's archives was brought to light by Dēmētrēs Papanikolaou in his book, where he shows its clear connection with the poem "Hidden Things."[19] I believe that the opposition to the laws ("'the wretched laws of society" / "whatever the rules may say, whatever the laws may say!") and the sense of community ("those who are made like me" / "like all women like herself") make the reflections of the schoolteacher Maria resonate with the two texts that most clearly express Cavafy's personal and social reflection on homosexuality. The intertextual kinship becomes even more pronounced if we add Cavafy's reference to the "more perfect society" in "Hidden Things," which meets the horizon of expectation of a sexually liberated society we find in Embiricos. It is almost certain that in the 1940s Embiricos was familiar neither with Cavafy's archive nor the so-called "hidden" poems, first published in 1968; this fact makes the affinity between their formulations even more profound, from a psychological standpoint.

Embiricos included Cavafy amongst his Beatified in *Oktana*, pairing him with the enigmatic "Aristarchus of Pleasures," who, according to Helena Badell's perceptive reading, is none other than Cavafy himself, the "grammarian of pleasures" from Alexandria.[20] There is no doubt that, in contrast to the general embarrassment around Cavafy's homosexuality, Embiricos admired Cavafy as a paradigm of the erotic poet, a bold celebrant of homosexual love. In my view, this is precisely why he includes him amongst the Beatified. This dimension is further underscored by the recordings of Giannēs Tsarouchēs' exquisite reading of Cavafy's poems, made at Embiricos' home in 1972.

Let us now turn to male homosexuality. *The Great Eastern* includes four episodes in which homosexual acts between men take place. Two occur on the ship itself, while the other two are embedded within the narrative—they take place in another space and time and are incorporated into the novel. Two involve strictly homosexual lovers, while the other two concern bisexual ones.

The central story is that of Czech violinist Jan Čerek and his young English lover, also a violinist, who is traveling disguised as a young woman and pretending to be the Czech violinist's niece (chapter 60). The two lovers are fleeing to escape the young man's family, who are searching for him in London, where the laws against male homosexuality are particularly severe. At one point during their lovemaking, the young homosexual fantasizes about an encounter with a phallic woman[21]—a figure that reappears in the analysis of Petros L.

The other three episodes are:

1. Pages from the diary of the Scottish writer MacGregor, which describe the homosexual relations of a young stable boy—first with his doctor and later with MacGregor himself (chapter 41).
2. Pages from an erotic novel in the English language read by the Canadian Flossie Norris, in which the sexual encounters of a homosexual Englishman with a postal messenger boy are described (chapter 64).
3. The description of a sexual encounter between physician-philosopher Hans Edelman with Russian-American boy Billy and female cabin attendant Betty (chapter 92).

"Officially Sanctioned Erotic Cohabitation Between Homosexuals Was Permitted, Under the Same Legal Provisions [as] Heterosexual Lovers"

Beyond these individual erotic scenes, however, and in order to understand how they fit within Embiricos' phenomenology of Eros, we must examine the place of homosexuality in his vision of a future, liberated world—in a "more perfect society," as Cavafy would have said—which echoes the famous utopia of Jules Verne, in the 61st chapter of *The Great Eastern*. In this future world, marriage has been abolished, and cohabitation of one or more lovers is permitted:

> Homosexuality, as follows from the foregoing, was not merely tolerated for both sexes, but officially sanctioned erotic cohabitation between homosexuals was permitted, under the same legal provisions governing the transfer of property and gifts between heterosexual lovers.

That is to say, there would exist a kind of civil union, exactly as for heterosexual couples, since marriage would have been abolished. It is striking that this was written shortly after the Second World War, during the very years when the British state imposed chemical castration on Alan Turing as an alternative sentence for the crime of homosexuality (1952).

And Jules Verne's utopian vision continues from where we left off:

> It must be emphasized, however, that although there still existed a fair number of exclusively homosexual individuals, complete homosexuality

> had far fewer adherents than in the past; and the censuses conducted every ten years, as well as the statistical studies, showed that those interested solely in erotic partners of their own sex had begun, over the last hundred or hundred and fifty years, to diminish steadily—whereas those same statistics showed the adherents of bisexuality (that is, those erotically interested in both sexes) to be multiplying in an inversely proportional manner.[22]

To understand this development, we must bear in mind that in the "future society" as described in Jules Verne's utopian vision, the taboo of incest will no longer exist.[23] With the eradication of the Oedipal complex, however, "Oedipal homosexuality"—that is, homosexuality arising from the boy's identification with the mother or the girl's attachment to the mother—will also have disappeared. Consequently, cases of strictly homosexual object choice will have been significantly reduced.

On the other hand, and again as a result of the eradication of the Oedipal complex, the strictly heterosexual orientation of object choice—arising from identification with father or mother—will likewise be diminished. Human beings will allow their bisexual nature to express itself freely. This explains the bisexual behavior of many characters in *The Great Eastern*, both men and women, among them the Scottish writer MacGregor and the Swiss physician-philosopher Hans Edelmann, both of whom are, in fact, personifications of Embiricos himself.

In Conclusion

I believe that the question of homosexuality particularly preoccupied Embiricos. Not because he was himself homosexual. From a psychoanalytic point of view, of course, he was, like us all, a latent bisexual, and, faithful to his own vision, he sought to transcend this in *The Great Eastern* by imagining even male homosexual scenes. The primary reason, however, for his special attention to homosexuality was that it represented the most intensely persecuted form of Eros. The sensitivity with which he turned towards this "erotic minority" (in the words of the schoolteacher Maria), in an era long before the demands of the modern LGBTQ+ movement, allows us to understand more clearly the ethical foundations of his emancipatory vision. This does not mean that Embiricos' vision perfectly coincides with the contemporary positions of that movement, which at times focuses particularly on the definition of "sexual identity." On the contrary, Embiricos invites us to rethink the question of sexual freedom without fixating on the question of identity, without replacing the old rigid boundaries between the sexes with new rigid categories of homosexual individuals.

In February 1940, in his text "Tektainomena" ("Events"), we encounter for the first time in his work the vision of "free libido," proposed as a counterweight to the sinister days Europe was living through after Hitler's invasion of Poland. This vision was presented as "a new reality, not only material, but also moral."[24] This vision is the source of the phenomenology of Eros to which Embiricos devoted much of his work in the following years. His erotic writings and the new reality they strive toward rest upon their own ethical premises. To grasp them, we must understand how deeply Embiricos had reflected on the relationship between the law and the freedom of Eros. The issue of homosexuality is emblematic in this respect. Equally groundbreaking for their time were his views on motherhood, contraception, and other related matters. Despite the enthusiasm that initially surrounded *The Great Eastern*, the phenomenology of Eros articulated by Embiricos has not been adequately understood in all its complexity, in its moral dimensions, and theoretical underpinnings. It is this gap that the present article seeks, at least in part, to fill.

Notes

1 Andreas Embiricos, "Hoi Horizontes ē hē phainomenologia tou erōtos," in *Hoi Kykloi tou Zōdiakou. Anekdota keimena apo tē syllogē "Grapta ē prosōpikē mythologia,"* ed. Giōrgēs Giatromanōlakēs (Athens: Agra, 2018), 35–42.
2 See Nikos Sigalas, "O Andreas Empeirikos anagnōstēs tou Breton, tou Frount kai tou Chenkel," *Synchrona Themata* no. 84 (2004): 45–53.
3 Nikos Sigalas, *O Andreas Embiricos kai ē istoria tou Ellēnikou Yperrealismou ē Brosta stēn ameiliktē archē tēs pragmatikotētas* (Athens: Agra, 2012), 211–223.
4 Etienne Balibar, "L'invention du surmoi: Freud et Kelsen 1922," in *Citoyen sujet et autres essais d'anthropologie philosophique* (Paris: Presses Universitaires de France, 2011), 383–434; and on the theory of the superego in the work of Embiricos, see Nikos Sigalas, *O Andreas Empeirikos kai . . .* (Paris: Presses Universitaires de France, 2011), 166–183.
5 Sigmund Freud, "Über die Psychogenese eines Falles von weiblicher Homosexualität," *Internationale Zeitschrift für Psychoanalyse* no. 6 (1920): 1–24. English translation: "The Psychogenesis of a Case of Homosexuality in a Woman," *S.E.*, vol. 18, 145ff.
6 See Élisabeth Roudinesco, "Psychanalyse et homosexualité: réflexions sur le désir pervers, l'injure et la fonction paternelle," *Cliniques méditerranéennes* no. 65 (2002): 7–34.
7 Sigmund Freud, *Eine Kindheitserinnerung des Leonardo da Vinci* (Leipzig und Wien: Deuticke Verlag, 1910); English translation: "Leonardo da Vinci and a Memory of His Childhood," *S.E.*, vol. 12, 59ff.
8 Cited in Roudinesco, "Psychanalyse et homosexualité: réflexions sur le désir pervers, l'injure et la fonction paternelle," *Cliniques méditerranéennes* no. 65 (2002): 7–34. English translation: Sigmund Freud, "Historical Notes: A Letter from Freud," *The American Journal of Psychiatry* 107, no. 10 (April 1951): 786–787.
9 Roudinesco, "Psychanalyse et homosexualité: réflexions sur le désir pervers, l'injure et la fonction paternelle," *Cliniques méditerranéennes* no. 65 (2002): 12.

10 Ch. 20, Embiricos used the term "*philhomophylia*" (same-sex love) in Greek in order to avoid the stigma attached to the standard Greek term "*homophylophilia*" (homosexuality), according to Vivika Empeirikou and Leōnidas Empeirikos. See Chapter 7 of the present volume.
11 Embiricos used the term "*philhomophylia*" (same-sex love) in Greek in order to avoid the stigma attached to the standard Greek term "*homophylophilia*" (homosexuality), according to Vivika Empeirikou and Leōnidas Empeirikos. See Chapter 7 of the present volume.
12 Translator's note: The reference properly corresponds to "The Ego and the Id," *S.E.*, vol. 19, 29.
13 Cf. Denys Ribas, "Formes de l'identification primitive à la mère," in *Identification* (Paris: PUF, 2002), 47–55.
14 Andreas Embiricos, "Anatolē," in *Hoi Kykloi tou Zōdiakou*, ed. Giōrgēs Giatromanōlakēs (Athens: Agra, 2018), 96–155.
15 Andreas Embiricos, "Anatolē," in *Hoi Kykloi tou Zōdiakou*, ed. Giōrgēs Giatromanōlakēs (Athens: Agra, 2018), 96–155.
16 Andreas Embiricos, "Anatolē," in *Hoi Kykloi tou Zōdiakou*, ed. Giōrgēs Giatromanōlakēs (Athens: Agra, 2018), 96–155.
17 Cited in full from Andreas Embiricos, "Anatolē," in *Hoi Kykloi tou Zōdiakou*, ed. Giōrgēs Giatromanōlakēs (Athens: Agra, 2018), 137.
18 Andreas Embiricos, *Ho Megas Anatolikos*, vol. 6 (Athens: Agra, 2011), 191.
19 Dēmētrēs Papanikolaou, *San ki'emena kamōmenoi: Ho homophylophilos Kavaphēs kai hē poiētikē tēs sexoualikotētas* (Athens: Ekdoseis Patakē, 2014).
20 Helena Badell Giralt, "Empeirikos, Kavafēs kai ē poiēsē tōn ēdonōn," *Nea Estia* no. 1744 (April 2002): 674–83.
21 Andreas Embiricos, *Ho Megas Anatolikos*, vol. 6, 136. Athens, Greece: AGRA Publications.
22 Cited in full from Andreas Embiricos, *Ho Megas Anatolikos*, vol. 6 (Athens: Agra, 2011), 172.
23 Savvas Michaēl, "O Andreas Empeirikos kai oi Thygateres tou Lōt," in *Plous kai kataplous tou "Megalou Anatolikou"* (Athens: Agra, 1995), 89–128; Nikos Sigalas, *O Andreas Empeirikos kai . . .* (Paris: Presses Universitaires de France, 2011), 189–91.
24 Andreas Embiricos, "Ta tektainomena," in *Hoi Kykloi tou Zōdiakou*, ed. Giōrgēs Giatromanōlakēs (Athens: Agra, 2018), 19–27.

Chapter 11

Marie Bonaparte and Andreas Embiricos

The Beginnings of Psychoanalysis in Greece. From Euphoria to Disillusionment

Leōnidas Embiricos[1]

In Memory of Marilia Aisenstein-Averoff

Leōnidas Embiricos gratefully acknowledges the assistance of Paraskeuas Matalas.

There is a limited amount of correspondence with Marie Bonaparte in the surviving papers of Andreas Embiricos. The most likely explanation for this is Embiricos' well-known reluctance when it came to letter writing, which, save for strictly practical matters, he engaged in sporadically even with his closest friends. This may also explain why Celia Bertin's biography of Marie Bonaparte made no mention of Andreas Embiricos, despite the fact that his friendship with her extended far beyond their psychoanalytic connection.[2]

By way of introduction, I refer the reader to the short biographical text on Marie Bonaparte [published in English translation in Chapter 5 of the present volume], which Embiricos wrote as an appendix to the Greek translation of her book *Identification of a Girl with Her Dead Mother*. The text was first published in the journal *Epoches* (nos. 6–8, 1963), republished by Agra Editions in Greek as a standalone volume in 1984, and later published in the present collection of Embiricos' psychoanalytic writings, also published in Greek by Agra in 2001.

This text illustrates the great importance Marie Bonaparte held for the Greek Psychoanalytic Group. The group was founded around the turn of 1949 to 1950, following interventions made personally by Marie Bonaparte at the *Société Psychanalytique de Paris* (SPP). It received recognition from the International Psychoanalytic Association with the support of other figures such as Glover, Anna Freud, and ultimately Ernest Jones. Thus, Marie Bonaparte played a decisive role in securing the establishment and international recognition of a group from a peripheral country. Both her status as a princess of Greece and her major institutional role within the SPP were decisive in making this possible. The group had initiated and planned to publish a series of psychoanalytic texts under the title *Publications of the Hellenic Psychoanalytic Group* [*Ekdoseis Hellēnikēs Psychanalytikēs Homados*], with translations undertaken not only by its three members, but outsiders as well. The group was intended to give way to the foundation of a Hellenic Psychoanalytic Society (once Frosso Karapanou completed her training analysis with Embiricos, which would give them the fourth member they were lacking), which would then become a component society of the International Psychoanalytic Association.

Such were the circumstances in 1949–50. In 1950, an intervention—which was most likely undertaken on the initiative of the Medical Association—was directed particularly against Andreas Embiricos, who was a non-physician psychoanalyst (lay analyst), and whom Marie Bonaparte, herself a lay analyst, defended in that capacity. This intervention led to Embiricos' resignation from the group in June 1951, the cessation of his analytic practice, and the dissolution of the Greek Psychoanalytic Group. Disheartened, Embiricos left for Paris immediately after the Amsterdam Psychoanalytical Congress in the summer of 1951, where he remained for three years. He maintained contact with the SPP, though he did not open a psychoanalytic practice in Paris, despite Bonaparte's encouragement to do so. Giōrgos Zavitzianos, after several moves, eventually settled in the United States and Canada, and joined the American Psychoanalytic Association; he returned to Greece only occasionally, discouraged by the impossibility of gaining official recognition for psychoanalysis in his homeland. Only Dēmētrēs Kouretas remained in Greece, without openly declaring his identity as a psychoanalyst, which he kept concealed behind his institutional role as a psychiatrist and later as a professor of psychiatry. Nonetheless, Marie Bonaparte continued to supervise his analytic work during this time.

The photograph that follows (Figure 11.1) constitutes a rare document attesting to Andreas Embiricos' participation in the 15th International Psychoanalytical Congress, held in Paris in 1938, which was organized thanks to the leadership and initiative of Marie Bonaparte. The photograph was recently discovered among Embiricos' papers and provides concrete evidence of his presence at that congress—something his close associates had long been aware of, yet which, in the absence of tangible proof, could previously only be cited as oral testimony.

Embiricos appears among the psychoanalysts attending the congress, several of whom were leading figures of the time. Notably present were Marie Bonaparte, Ernest Jones, and Edouard Pichon. The latter had recently become president of the SPP, yet was aligned with the nationalistic, royalist, and anti-Semitic organization *Action Française*. He may have been, at least in part, responsible for the suicide of Jean-Frois Wittmann, a leftist Jewish painter associated with the Surrealist group, a psychoanalyst, and close friend of Andreas Embiricos, who, five years earlier, had introduced Embiricos to André Breton.

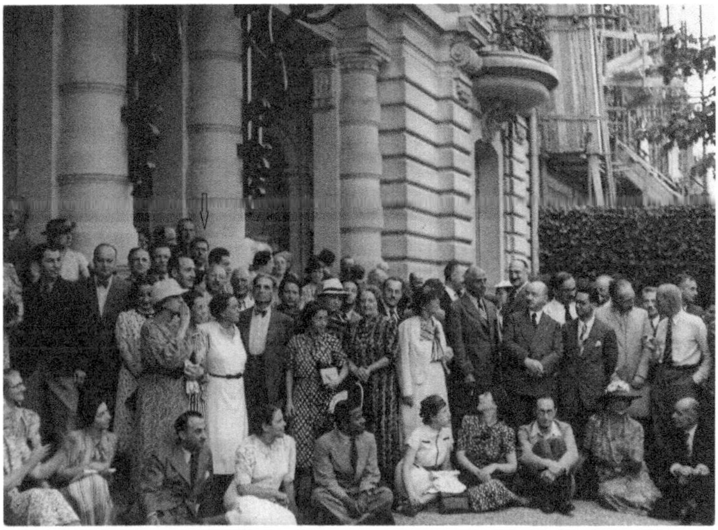

Figure 11.1 Photograph from the 15th International Psychoanalytical Congress, Paris (August 1938). Seated at the lower right (second from the right) is Marie Bonaparte. Andreas Embiricos is visible standing at the rear left, beneath the arrow. Immediately to his right stands Jacques Lacan, with whom Embiricos had been acquainted since the 1930s, the two being connected through their mutual involvement with Surrealism.

In what follows, I reproduce a letter from Wittmann to Embiricos, dated February 1936:

Bien cher ami,

Merci infiniment de la charmante surprise—ce joli porte-cigarettes que Simon Georgiades nous a remis de votre part. J'ai porté le sien à Laforgue qui en a été enchanté; et qui a dû vous remercier lui-même. Georgiades nous a dit que vous avez pris un de ses amis en analyse, je l'ai dit à Laforgue, et nous vous félicitons tous deux. Vous êtes certainement très doué pour comprendre le langage de l'inconscient, et j'espère que vous pourrez mener cette cure à bien.

Ici, rien de très nouveau: on attend le résultat des élections de Mai prochain, en se réjouissant des magnifiques élections espagnoles, et du sérieux sénateur communiste que le Front populaire vient de faire passer hier en remplacement du vieux Laval! Vous voyez que nous avons toutes les raisons d'être optimistes en ce moment—à condition d'ailleurs de redoubler d'efforts car la réaction ne désarme pas.

Je pense que vous avez les bonnes nouvelles d'André Breton. Il paraît qu'il va bien et élève son enfant en père excellent.

Mille souvenirs amicaux de Josée et de
Jean Frois-Wittman. Le 21 fév. 1936.

[My very dear friend,

Many thanks for the delightful surprise—the lovely cigarette case that Simon Georgiades delivered to us on your behalf. I took Laforgue's to him, and he was delighted; he must have thanked you himself. Georgiades told us that you have taken one of his friends into analysis; I mentioned it to Laforgue, and we both congratulate you. You are certainly very gifted at understanding the language of the unconscious, and I hope you will be able to carry this treatment through successfully.

Here, nothing particularly new: we are waiting for the results of the upcoming May election,[3] rejoicing meanwhile at the splendid elections in Spain,[4] and at the very serious Communist senator the Popular Front was able to seat as a replacement for old Laval![5] You see, we have every reason to be optimistic at the moment—provided, of course, that we redouble our efforts, for the reactionary forces are not backing down.

I imagine you have good news from André Breton. It seems that he is doing well and is raising his child as an excellent father.

A thousand friendly regards from Josée and
Jean-Frois Wittmann. 21 Feb., 1936.[6]]

At the 15th Paris Congress, Andreas Embiricos was expecting—as Marie Bonaparte had promised him—to meet Freud, provided the latter's health allowed him to travel from London. Freud, only a few months earlier after having been rescued from the Nazis by Marie Bonaparte and Ernest Jones, was scheduled to read his new metapsychological text, *Der Mann Moses*, or a part of it.[7] In the end, it was his daughter Anna who read the paper, as Freud himself was unable to attend. Embiricos' reading of the published text a year later was one of the principal inspirations behind his own work *Ta Tektainomena* [*The Events*].[8]

The next photograph (Figure 11.2) is from the International Psychoanalytical Congress held in Zurich in 1949—the first International Psychoanalytical Congress after the Second World War. It shows Andreas Embiricos, Vivika Empeirikou, and Dēmētrēs Kouretas. In the following photograph (Figure 11.3), also taken at the same Congress, Marie Bonaparte appears in the center, with Andreas Embiricos to her right.

In these two photographs, preserved among the papers of Andreas Embiricos, appear many of the leading figures of psychoanalysis during the years 1938 to 1949—that is, before and after the war and the Nazi occupation, and before and after Freud's death. Among them are Max Eitingon, one of the

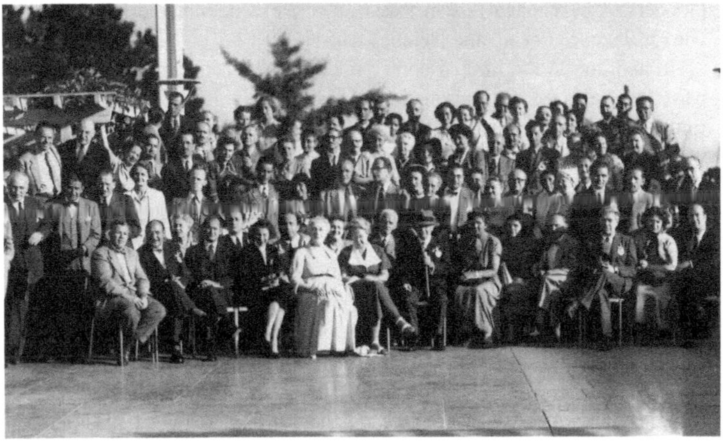

Figure 11.2 Photograph from the International Psychoanalytical Congress in Zurich, 1949. In the front row, seated on the right (from right to left), are Giōrgios Zavitzianos, Vivika Empeirikou, and Andreas Embiricos. Standing directly behind Embiricos is Dēmētrēs Kouretas.

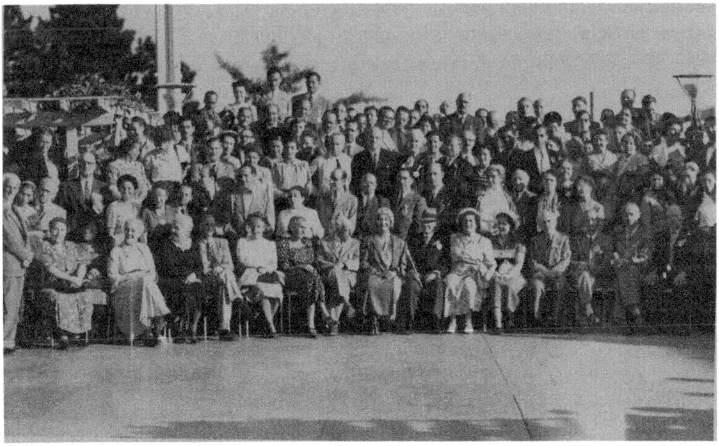

Figure 11.3 Photograph from the Psychoanalytical Congress in Zurich, 1949. Seated at the center is Marie Bonaparte. Standing, second from right, is Andreas Embiricos, with Vivika Empeirikou beside him.

pioneers of psychoanalysis in Russia, Anna Freud, Melanie Klein, Edward Glover, Jacques Lacan, and Helene Deutsch.

In addition to the limited correspondence between Embiricos and Bonaparte, we have the inscriptions in the books that Marie Bonaparte gifted to Embiricos, as well as her evident and ongoing efforts to protect him—efforts which, to our great surprise, did not begin after the Second World War but as early as 1937. From Embiricos' surviving papers, studied by Nikos Sigalas, we obtain several important pieces of information. Sigalas precisely identifies Bonaparte and Embiricos' first meeting as having taken place on 6 April 1937. Embiricos opened his psychoanalytic practice after consulting with René Laforgue and members of the Paris Psychoanalytic Society. He had undergone an analysis with Laforgue from 1927 to 1931 and later pursued a training analysis with him, including supervision, regularly traveling from Athens to Paris from December 1935 onward. Embiricos' practice was the first officially recognized psychoanalytic practice in Athens. From the outset, his intent, and indeed his urgency, in wanting to establish a society in coordination with the SPP was to stymie the influence of the Jungians, whose presence in Greece was stronger at the time.

We have thus discovered something previously unknown: that Embiricos and Bonaparte became acquainted in April 1937, in the midst of the Metaxas dictatorship and the 4th of August Regime. Marie Bonaparte had by then returned to Greece, officially as a princess of the royal house, following the November 1935 plebiscite. The "so very democratic princess of ours," as Embiricos would later call her, sent him a letter on 4 April 1937, through her secretary Kornēlia Palē, inviting him to pay her a call, having learned from the SPP and Laforgue himself that there was a practicing psychoanalyst in Athens:

Sir,

Her Royal Highness the Princess George of Greece wishes to receive you in audience on Tuesday the 6th of this month at a quarter past seven.

Kornēlia Palē.[9]

Laforgue had already written to Embiricos, informing him that Princess Marie would be coming to Athens in eight days and wished to meet him. Up to that point, Embiricos had moved within two intersecting but distinct circles: the Surrealist and the psychoanalytic. In 1935, he had actively introduced Surrealism to Greece and maintained a close friendship and direct collaboration with the major poet, essayist, and critic known today as Nikolas Kalas, but who was then still known as Nikos Kalamarēs or Nikēta Rantos.[10]

His meeting with Marie Bonaparte in 1937, however, marked the beginning of the rupture between Embiricos and Kalamarēs, owing to the latter's sharp opposition to the Greek royal family. As Nikos Sigalas' remarkably lucid reconstruction of the sequence of events shows, the break was not immediate, yet it led to a lasting estrangement between the two men and to the stagnation of efforts to consolidate Surrealism as a movement in Greece. The disagreement was both personal and political, but it also concerned their divergent interpretations of psychoanalytic theory and its concepts, and of their applicability to political action—specifically, to anti-Fascist engagement. Thus emerges a paradox: 1937 stands as the apex of Embiricos' Surrealist activities, undertaken by a man entirely opposed to the monarchy in Greece, yet this coincides with his fervent and sustained efforts to secure the institutional establishment of psychoanalysis in the country. In this endeavor, he was aided by none other than Princess Marie of Greece, who had returned to the country following the royalist plebiscite.

In his effort to institutionalize psychoanalysis through the mediation of Marie Bonaparte, Embiricos wrote a letter, as suggested by Marie Bonaparte following the 1938 Paris Congress, to Alexandros Koryzēs, then Minister of Public Health and Welfare, who would later become prime minister and take his own life on 19 April 1941 during the German invasion of Athens. He wrote to him, as follows, on 16 December 1938:

> That permission be granted for the establishment of a Hellenic Psychoanalytic Society, composed of *qualified* members, whether physicians or not. The Society shall train, through its members, those who wish to practice the profession of psychoanalyst, and shall regulate all psychoanalytic matters in the country as the Greek branch of the International Psychoanalytic Association. Given that no authority currently exists in Greece to oversee those who identify themselves as psychoanalysts, it should be permitted—until the foundation and organization of the Hellenic Psychoanalytic Society—for the profession to be practiced by persons whose specific psychoanalytic competence has been recognized by foreign psychoanalysts or psychoanalytic institutes abroad.[11]

This letter appears never to have received a reply, as no trace of one has been found among Embiricos' papers. More importantly, this is confirmed by the testimony of Vivika, the woman who would later become Embiricos' wife, who heard it directly from him at a time close to the events in question.

An important document attesting to Embiricos' gratitude for the events preceding the War and the Occupation is the draft of a letter he addressed to Marie Bonaparte on 26 January 1940:

Altesse,

Veuillez me permettre de vous remercier encore une fois et de tout mon cœur pour votre grande bienveillance à mon égard, ainsi que pour l'aide précieuse que vous avez bien voulu m'accorder durant votre séjour à Athènes, pour lesquels je vous serai toujours profondément reconnaissant. Nous vous souhaitons, ma fiancée et moi, un bon voyage.

A. L. Embiricos[12]

[Your Highness,

Allow me once again, and with all my heart, to thank you for your great kindness toward me, as well as for the invaluable assistance you so graciously offered me during your stay in Athens, for which I shall forever remain deeply grateful. My fiancée and I wish you a pleasant journey.

A. L. Embiricos]

The "hardships, misunderstandings, misrepresentations, slander, and hostility," as Embiricos writes in the text I cited at the beginning, continued to be directed against him, and redoubled after the war, between 1945 and 1946. It was only when, once again through a plebiscite on the monarchy, in September 1946, Marie Bonaparte returned to Greece that these hostilities seem to have subsided somewhat, at least for a time. They concerned not only Embiricos' status as a non-medical psychoanalyst, but also opposition to the formal establishment of a psychoanalytic institution, and later to the very existence of the Greek Psychoanalytic Group, affiliated with the SPP, as well as to the founding of a Hellenic Psychoanalytic Society. The intervention of the Municipal Police in Athens in 1950, directed specifically against Embiricos, is indicative that the authorities themselves (perhaps even the Royal Palace) were opposed to such an establishment, despite Marie Bonaparte's influence.

When the arrangement was made for the publication of Andreas Embiricos' psychoanalytic writings with the late Thanasēs Tzavaras—who restored Embiricos' reputation as a psychoanalyst, indeed as the foremost psychoanalyst in Greece—he refused to give credence to the statements of Vivika Empeirikou and others in Embiricos' close circle, who maintained that Embiricos had been informally prohibited by the police from practicing psychoanalysis, under threat of prosecution for the "practice of an unlicensed profession." His skepticism was strengthened due to his inability to locate any reference, even an internal memo, to such an intervention in the police archives. Moreover, Lena Atzina, then a student of Tzavaras and a historian of psychoanalysis herself, found no trace in any of the accessible records of the Municipal Police of the repeated visits by police officers seeking to force the closure of his psychoanalytic practice in 1950.[13]

The fact that no formal charges were ever brought was likely due to the social prestige of the Embiricos name. A more discreet approach was adopted, one that would leave no trace of either the complainant or the police, and that would avoid provoking public scandal. It was probably in this tacit manner that Embiricos was granted the six-month period he himself had requested in order to gradually terminate with his patients before closing his practice permanently in June 1951.

However, given that the threat of prosecution had been verbal, Thanasēs Tzavaras lacked any tangible proof of the pressure Embiricos was under to close his practice and did not find the oral testimony regarding this episode convincing. The only witnesses were members of Embiricos' immediate circle: Dēmētrēs Kouretas and his wife Antonia, Giōrgos Zavitzianos, and above all, Vivika Empeirikou, who was an eyewitness. I myself had a long conversation with Giōrgos Zavitzianos on this matter in the 1980s and asked him to record his testimony and recollections of this event in writing. However, he never managed to do so. Thus, for many years, a false rumor persisted: that Embiricos had not been a legitimate psychoanalyst, that he had supposedly been denounced by his own patients (which never occurred), and, secondly, that his interests had simply led him in other directions. In this way, Embiricos' name was nearly erased from the history of psychoanalysis in Greece. Although Tzavaras, through his research, restored Embiricos' to his rightful position within the Greek psychoanalytic milieu, refuted these rumors, and rightly connected Embiricos' literary production of those years with his psychoanalytic activity, during which free associations from the couch nourished the flow of his writing, he nonetheless formulated the following conclusion regarding Embiricos' cessation of his psychoanalytic practice: that "literature won him over."[14]

I believe that Tzavaras was mistaken on this point, for not only did literature not "win him over," but the cessation of psychoanalytic practice also brought his writing, whether prose, poetry, or essays, to a complete halt for at least six years. It was only after 1956 that he began to write again, and then exclusively autobiographical texts for an unfinished "Personal Encyclopedia" [*Prosōpikē Enkyklopaideia*], produced while in a state of depression and withdrawal from public life. Only after 1958, and especially from 1960 onward, did he compose his major collections *Oktana* and *Hē Sēmeron ōs Aurion kai ōs Chthes* [*Today as Tomorrow and Yesterday*]. If any art "won him over," it was photography, which he practiced with great skill and technical mastery, though his photographs only ever appeared once in public, at the photographic exhibition held at the "Ilisos" gallery in 1956.

Embiricos' relationship with Marie Bonaparte continued long after the end of their psychoanalytic association, indeed, until her death, and even grew warmer in Athens, Paris, Saint-Cloud, and Saint-Tropez, at her villa *Le Lys de mer*.

The next photograph [Figure 11.4] shows Marie Bonaparte, photographed by Andreas Embiricos during a friendly visit in the garden of her home in Saint-Tropez in the 1950s. In the adjacent photograph [Figure 11.5], Marie Bonaparte is seen in 1955, again photographed by Andreas Embiricos at her residence in Saint-Cloud.

The small body of correspondence from this period following the cessation of Embiricos' psychoanalytic practice was provided to Tzavaras, who made use of it in his writings on the relationship between Andreas Embiricos

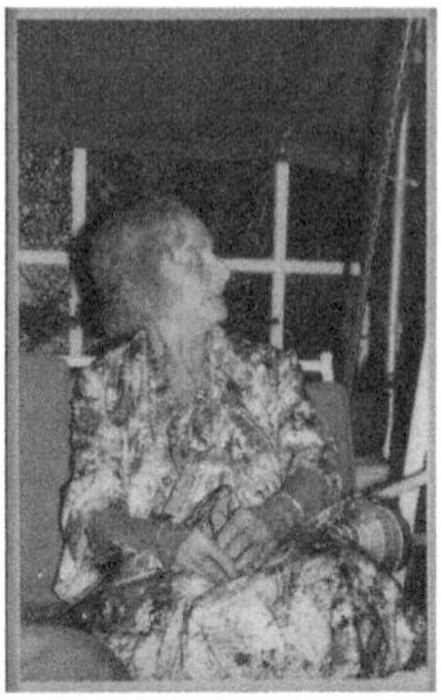

Figure 11.4 Marie Bonaparte photographed by Andreas Embiricos at her home in Saint-Tropez.

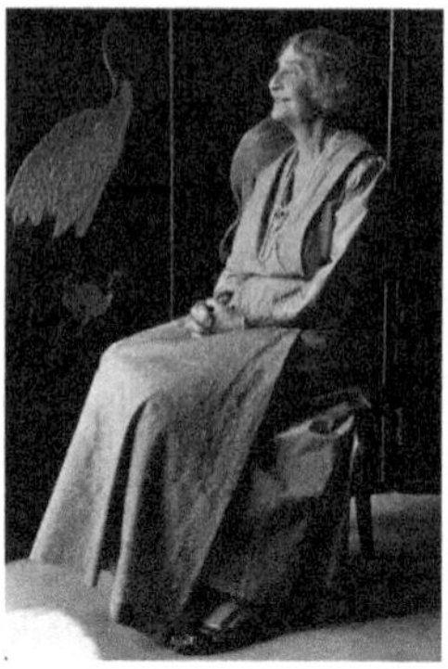

Figure 11.5 Marie Bonaparte, photographed by Andreas Embiricos in 1955 at her home in Saint-Cloud.

and Marie Bonaparte. These letters concern, first, Bonaparte's moral support for Embiricos, who had fallen into depression during the Amsterdam Psychoanalytical Congress as a result of being forced to shut down his analytic practice. All of Bonaparte's letters are very warm and invariably begin with *Mon cher ami* [My dear friend]. Another part of this brief correspondence consists of Bonaparte's proposal to hire Embiricos as her personal secretary, should a Third World War break out, because, with the globalization of the Korean War, they might have been compelled to relocate to America, where neither Embiricos nor Bonaparte, both lay analysts, could have practiced psychoanalysts.

At that time, the fear of a global—and indeed nuclear—war was part of daily life, owing to Douglas MacArthur's threat to use nuclear weapons against China, as the army of the victorious Chinese Revolution invaded South Korea following the American landing at Incheon. We now know that Harry Truman ultimately prevented him from doing so. During that crisis, Embiricos' relationship with Marie Bonaparte ceased to be primarily psychoanalytic; it became particularly friendly, with literature at its center, but always against the backdrop of psychoanalysis.

Embiricos dedicated two texts from his *Grapta* [*Writings*] to Marie Bonaparte. The first, "Hermolaos the Macedonian," bears the dedication: "To H.R.H. Princess Marie of Greece," and the second, "Oedipus Rex," is dedicated "To Marie Bonaparte." Embiricos thus made this double dedication in acknowledgment of her two statuses. As Michalēs Chrysanthopoulos has insightfully analyzed, the latter, and more intimate, of the two dedications, has as its background their possible discussions regarding the centrality of the Oedipus complex and the corresponding concept of the latency period in psychoanalysis.[15] Embiricos was a supporter of Malinowski's positions in *The Sexual Life of Savages in North-Western Melanesia* (which he read in its 1930 French translation), concerning the non-universality of the Oedipus complex and the latency period, or at least the impossibility of directly applying them outside the Euro-Asiatic cultural framework.[16] Marie Bonaparte, however, although she agreed with Malinowski's conclusions to some extent, also participated in funding Géza Róheim's major expedition, which resulted in a work contrary to Malinowski's theses: *The Riddle of the Sphinx*.[17] According to Chrysanthopoulos, the hypothetical discussions—or possible disagreements, voiced or unvoiced—between Embiricos and Bonaparte are inscribed in this dedication and reveal Embiricos' ideological position: his expectation of a future, post-Oedipal humanity, which Chrysanthopoulos terms Embiricos' post-Oedipal or post-psychoanalytic utopia. This position makes him appear to diverge from Freudian orthodoxy on this point. Yet, as he constantly expresses through his writings, Embiricos remained entirely faithful to Freudian doctrine with respect to the present day, adopting an explicitly anti-Jungian stance. This metapsychological vision, this expectation that defines the horizon of Embiricos' thought after the Second World War, derives entirely from psychoanalysis, from which, as he writes elsewhere, he awaits "with unshakeable certainty, the coming of man's maturity."[18]

In the text "Oedipus Rex," the materiality and corporeality of the incestuous desire constitute an explicitly anti-Jungian allusion. The dedication "To Marie Bonaparte" simultaneously signals the solidarity of the two in their shared opposition to Jung's desexualization of the unconscious, and, in particular, of the Oedipus complex.[19]

This topic was first explored by Michalēs Chrysanthopoulos in his paper "Personal Mythology and Psychoanalytical Theory in Andreas Empeirikos," presented at the conference organized in Athens in October 2006 by the *Association Internationale de l'histoire de la Psychanalyse* and the Hellenic Society for Psychoanalytic Psychotherapy.

The conservative leadership of French psychoanalysis under Sacha Nacht prevented Embiricos from expressing himself as freely as he wished in his effort to become a full member (from *membre affilié* to *membre adhérent*) of the SPP with his 1950 paper published in the *Revue Française de Psychanalyse* (Chapter 1 of the present volume). Marie Bonaparte, by contrast, allowed for considerable theoretical latitude, at least in their discussions.[20]

The visits Embiricos and his wife made to Marie Bonaparte in Paris, Saint-Tropez, and Athens, as well as the excursions they took together in Greece, are documented in photographs and 16mm film footage. Excerpts from these were included in three documentaries: Tasos Psarras' on Embiricos (2003) for Ilias Giannakakis' series *Epoches kai Syngrapheis* [*Seasons and Writers*]; by the same director in 2009, for the *Paraskēnio* [*Backstage*] series, entitled *Andreas Empeirikos, o poiētēs mesa apo tis eikones tou* [*Andreas Embiricos: The Poet Through His Own Images*]; and by Giōrgos Skeuas for a *Paraskēnio* documentary on Marie Bonaparte.

During one of his visits to Marie Bonaparte's home on Akadēmias Street, Embiricos brought his tape recorder and recorded a lengthy conversation between them about Nikos Kazantzakis, whom she greatly admired. She supported his candidacy for the Nobel Prize and defended him against the threatened excommunication by the Greek Orthodox Church. At the beginning of the recording, Marie Bonaparte is heard joking: "*Monsieur Embiricos est un homme dangereux parce qu'il a amené ce machin-là . . .*" ("Monsieur Embiricos is a dangerous man because he has brought this contraption [the tape recorder]"). A portion of this recording can be heard in Giōrgos Skevas' *Paraskēnio* documentary on Marie Bonaparte.

Embiricos' relationship with Marie Bonaparte through literature also included his translation of her literary work *Les Glauques Aventures de Flyda des Mers*. This translation has remained unpublished, as from the 1950s onward Embiricos did not publish any further work, apart from *Grapta ē Prosōpikē Mythologia* [*Writings or Personal Mythology*], which he himself censored before its 1960 publication. Marie Bonaparte, for her part, gifted him all of her books, inscribed to him. One of these dedications reads: "*au collègue qui fut le pionnier de la psychanalyse en Grèce, à l'écrivain aux couleurs éclatantes, et à l'ami*" ["to the colleague who was the pioneer of psychoanalysis in Greece, to the writer with brilliant colors, and to the friend"] (see Figures 11.6–11.8). From the first of these dedications, it also appears that Embiricos had translated another of her literary works, *Le Printemps sur mon Jardin*, though that translation has not been found among his papers.

Another aspect of the close relationship that developed between them during the 1950s is revealed when Marie Bonaparte decided to donate the enormous library of her father, Prince Roland Bonaparte. She invited Embiricos to first choose whichever books he wished from it. Today, Embiricos' library includes the multivolume *Géographie Universelle* by the anarchist geographer Élisée Reclus, along with many other works that bear, on the inside of their hard covers, a printed label with the prince's scholarly ex libris: *Bibliothèque du Prince Roland Bonaparte* (Figure 11.9).

After ending his psychoanalytic practice, as mentioned above, Embiricos devoted himself almost exclusively to photography for at least six years, and he continued this activity until the end of his life. He channeled into photography the same passion he had once invested in psychoanalysis and his efforts to institutionalize it in Greece. The two photographs of Marie Bonaparte presented here belong to this body of photographic

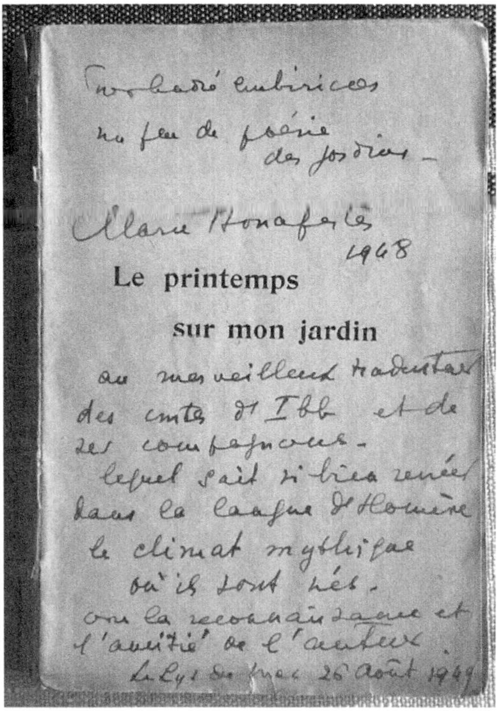

Figure 11.6 "Pour André Embiricos un peu de poésie des jardins. Marie Bonaparte 1948. Au merveilleux traducteur des contes d'Ibb et de ses compagnons, lequel sait si bien recréer dans la langue d'Homère le climat mythique où ils sont nés. Avec la reconnaissance et l'amitié de l'auteur. Le Lys de mer, 26 août 1949."

["For Andreas Embiricos, a bit of garden poetry. Marie Bonaparte, 1948. To the marvelous translator of the tales of Ibb and his companions, who knows so well how to recreate, in the language of Homer, the mythical atmosphere in which they were born. With the author's gratitude and friendship. *Le Lys de mer*, 26 August 1949."]

In: Marie Bonaparte, *Le Printemps sur mon Jardin* (Paris: Flammarion, 1924).

work and represent only a small part, not only of his photographic production as a whole, but also of the many snapshots and portraits he took of Marie Bonaparte.

One year after the death of Marie Bonaparte, Embiricos wrote an exceptionally moving text in her memory, which forms Chapter 4 of the present volume.

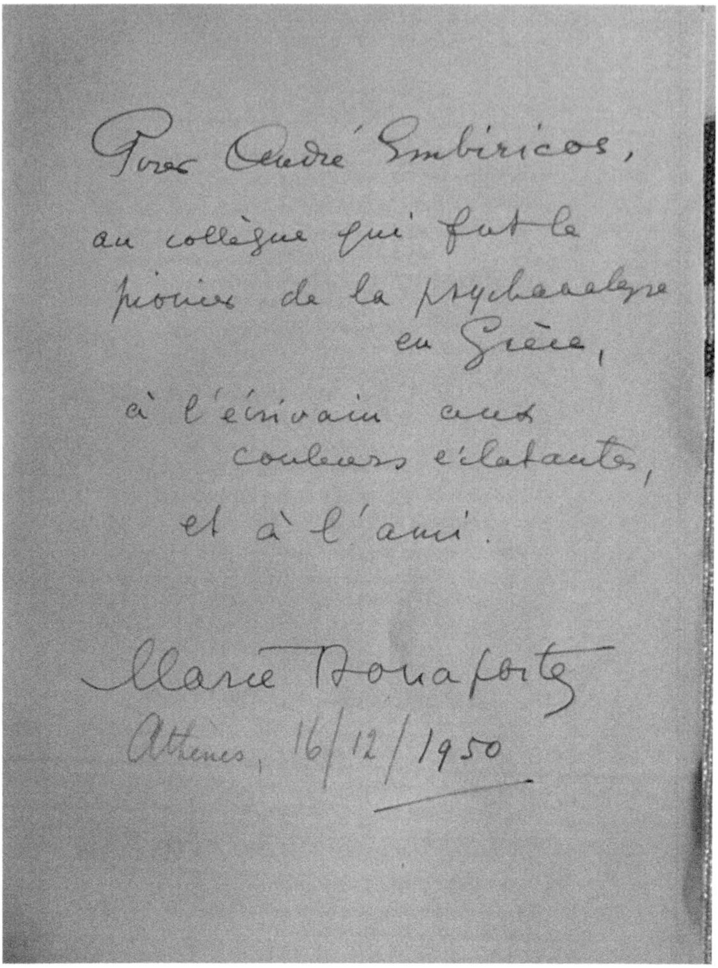

Pour André Embiricos,
au collègue qui fut le
pionnier de la psychanalyse
en Grèce,
à l'écrivain aux
couleurs éclatantes,
et à l'ami.

Marie Bonaparte
Athènes, 16/12/1950

Figure 11.7 "Pour André Embiricos, au collègue qui fut le pionnier de la psychanalyse en Grèce, à l'écrivain aux couleurs éclatantes, et à l'ami. Marie Bonaparte. Athènes, 16/12/1950."

["For Andreas Embiricos, to the colleague who was the pioneer of psychoanalysis in Greece, to the writer with brilliant colors, and to the friend. Marie Bonaparte. Athens, 16 Dec. 1950."]

In: Marie Bonaparte, *Les Glanes des Jours* (London: Imago, 1950).

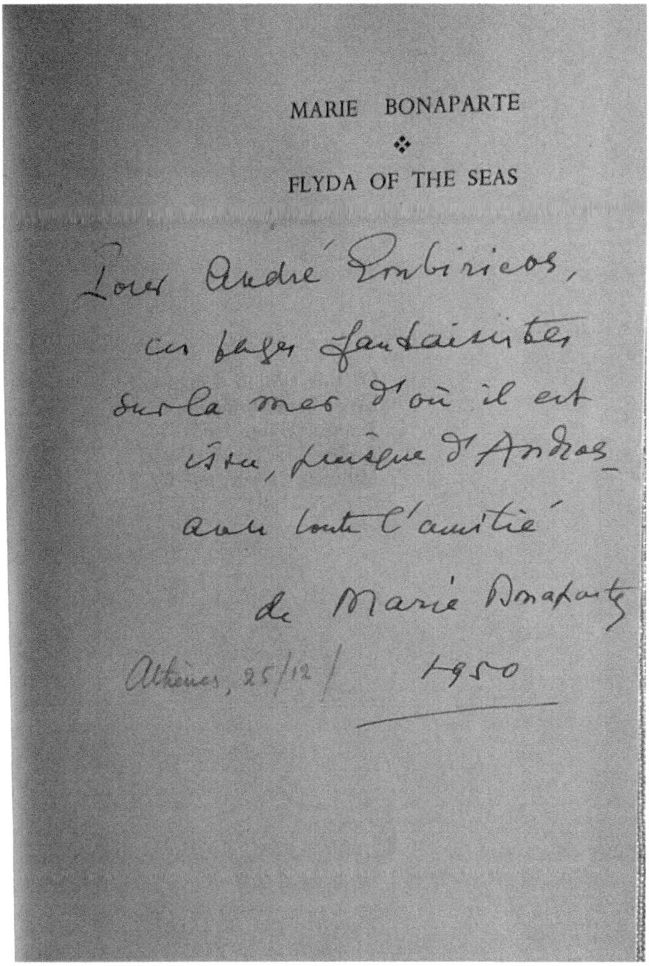

Figure 11.8 "Pour André Embircos, ces pages fantaisistes sur la mer d'où il est venu, puisque d'Andros, avec toute l'amitié de Marie Bonaparte. Athènes, 25/12/1950."

["For Andreas Embiricos, these fanciful pages about the sea whence he came, since he is from Andros, with all the friendship of Marie Bonaparte. Athens, 25 Dec. 1950."]

In: Marie Bonaparte, *Flyda of the Seas* (London: Imago, 1950).

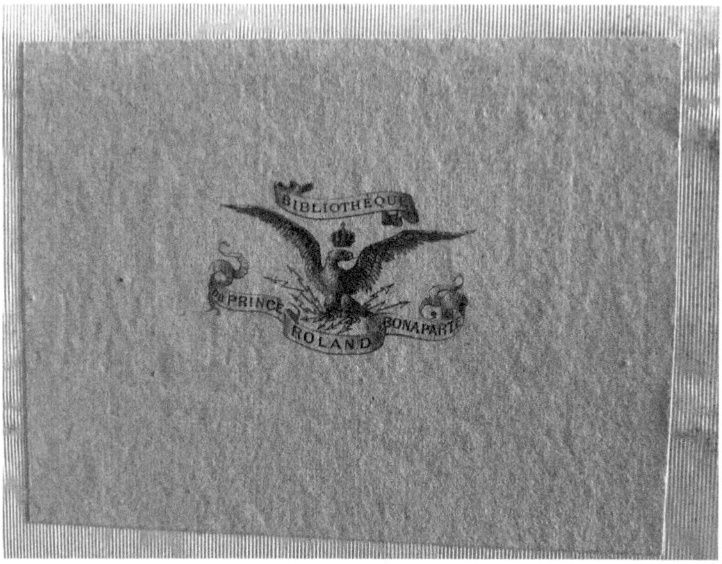

Figure 11.9 The *ex libris* of Marie Bonaparte's father, Roland, on the copy of Élisée Reclus' *La Terre: Description des Phénomènes de la Vie du Globe* (1872), which Marie Bonaparte gave to Andreas Embiricos.

Notes

1 Leonidas Embiricos is a historian.
2 Celia Bertin, *La Dernière Bonaparte* (Paris: Perrin, 1982).
3 The French elections were scheduled to take place on 26 April and 3 May 1936. They would result in the great victory of the Popular Front and the election of Léon Blum as Prime Minister.
4 In the elections that happened five months before this letter was written, on 16 February 1936, the Spanish left Popular Front came to power, a fact that would lead, a few months later, to the military coup and the Spanish Civil War.
5 On 23 February, elections were held for the Senate seat representing the Department of the Seine, resulting in the victory of the Communist candidate of the Popular Front, Jean-Marie Clamamus. The seat had previously been held by Pierre Laval (1883–1945), who had served as prime minister until January 1936 and who would again become prime minister during the period of the German occupation. After the war, he was sentenced to death for having collaborated with the Nazis.
6 This letter was published in: Nikos Sigalas, *Ho Andreas Empeirikos kai hē historia tou hellēnikou hyperrealismou. Ē brosta stēn ameiliktē archē tēs pragmatikotētas* (Athens: Agra, 2012), 332.

7 English translation: "Moses and Monotheism," in *Standard Edition of the Complete Psychological Works of Sigmund Freud*, vol. 23, ed. and trans. James Strachey (London: Hogarth, 1964), 1–140.
8 Andreas Empeirikos, *Hoi Kykloi tou Zōdiakou: Anekdota keimena apo tē syllogē "Grapta ē prosōpikē mythologia"* (Athens: Agra, 2018), 19–27.
9 Nikos Sigalas, *Ho Andreas Empeirikos kai hē historia tou hellēnikou hyperrealismou. Ē brosta stēn ameiliktē archē tēs pragmatikotētas* (Athens: Agra, 2012), 234.
10 Nikos Sigalas, *Ho Andreas Empeirikos kai hē historia tou hellēnikou hyperrealismou. Ē brosta stēn ameiliktē archē tēs pragmatikotētas* (Athens: Agra, 2012), 234.
11 Nikos Sigalas, *Ho Andreas Empeirikos kai hē historia tou hellēnikou hyperrealismou. Ē brosta stēn ameiliktē archē tēs pragmatikotētas* (Athens: Agra, 2012), 338.
12 Nikos Sigalas, *Ho Andreas Empeirikos kai hē historia tou hellēnikou hyperrealismou. Ē brosta stēn ameiliktē archē tēs pragmatikotētas* (Athens: Agra, 2012), 337.
13 Lena Atzina, *Hē makra eisagōgē tēs psychanalysēs stēn Hellada: Psychanalytes, iatrikoi thesmoi kai koinōnikes proslēpseis, 1910–1990* (Athens: Exantas, 2004).
14 See Chapter 8 of the present volume.
15 Michalēs Chrysanthopoulos, "Personal Mythology and Psychoanalytical Theory in Andreas Empeirikos" (paper presented at the conference of the *Association Internationale de l'histoire de la Psychanalyse* and the Hellenic Society for Psychoanalytic Psychotherapy, Athens, October 2006).
16 Bronisław Malinowski, *La vie sexuelle des sauvages du nord-ouest de la Mélanésie* (Paris: Payot, 1930).
17 Géza Roheim, *The Riddle of the Sphinx* (London: Hogarth, 1934).
18 Andreas Embiricos, *Hoi Kykloi tou Zōdiakou: Anekdota keimena apo tē syllogē "Grapta ē prosōpikē mythologia"* (Athens: Agra, 2018), 206.
19 Michalēs Chrisanthopoulos, *Hekato chronia perasan kai hena karavi: ho hellēnikos hyperrealismos kai hē kataskeuē tēs paradosēs* (Athens: Agra, 2012), 317–327.
20 Brigitte Lemérer, "Andréas Embiricos: psychanalyse et surréalisme," *Essaim* no. 10 (2002): 129–132.